The ~~Cost~~ Price of Having A Baby

CA Aarti Tibrewala Darooka

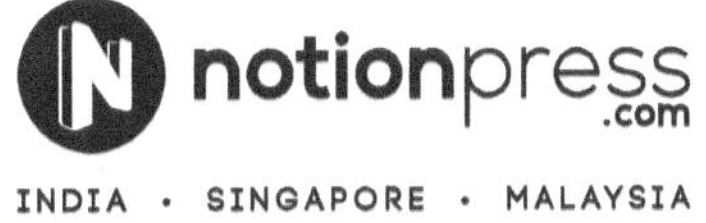

INDIA · SINGAPORE · MALAYSIA

ISBN 979-8-89277-945-6

CONTENTS

Introduction..5

Chapter 1:   Communication and Consent 11

Chapter 2:   Timing..20

Chapter 3:   Carrying Your Career Along with the Baby.............36

Chapter 4:   Space for the Baby 43

Chapter 5:   Basic Biology of Becoming Pregnant........................49

Chapter 6:   Conditioning The Mind 55

Chapter 7:   The Family Support System 61

Chapter 8:   The Backup Mechanism 71

Chapter 9:   The Conception Process...80

Chapter 10:   Preparing Your Finances for the Pregnancy 85

Chapter 11:   Problems In Conception...94

Chapter 12:   Physical Fitness and Pregnancy................................100

Chapter 13: Physical Fitness for the other Parent.........................106

Chapter 14: The Emotional Burden of Wanting to Get
Pregnant...112

Chapter 15: How to Deal With the Irritants................................121

Chapter 16: Plan B 129

Chapter 17: Discretionary Listening Through the Pregnancy...134

Chapter 18: Delivery..140

Chapter 19: What It Costs to Raise a Child................................147

Chapter 20: Dealing With The Newborn and The New Mom ..155

Chapter 21: Important Notes for The First Few Days
After Child Birth 162

Chapter 22: Post-partum Blues 169

Chapter 23: Plan C...175

INTRODUCTION

First came the cries, and then came the little face, blinking eyes trying to adjust to the light. These were her first moments in the real world, after all. I was barely conscious, but I reached out to the tiny fingers. They quickly curled around my index finger, not quite going all around it. They were a little clammy, maybe from being in the womb full of fluid. I thought she didn't want to let go. But before I could do anything about it, I slipped into a deep sleep. When I came to, my first thought was of the little fingers. This is how I met my baby.

Human beings foster a wide range of feelings, ranging from love, hatred and care to selfishness, among others. The strongest of such feelings is the yearning of a newborn for her mother. It is so natural and so deep that it can never be mitigated by any other presence. The bond between the child and her parent is the first ever a human being forms—the nourishment she derives from her mother's body, even in the womb, can't be received from elsewhere. It is the only bond in which surrender and love are complete and without question. The loyalty is unquestionable, and the relationship is permanent. It is no wonder, therefore, that the bond between a parent and child is considered the most unadulterated form of love.

Many argue that there is a growing number of people who see parenthood as a process not meant for them. A lot of my own friends have either figured that having a baby, with or without thinking about marriage, is not something they want. A lot of these people also feel that being a 'pet parent' is more than enough commitment. For a few others, there is either no love for children, or they feel that kids lead to too much preoccupation that distracts from their goals, ambitions, and right to live life to the fullest. Some people like ace entrepreneur Nikhil Kamath don't believe in having children to create a legacy for his family and don't necessarily want to ruin, to quote Kamath, "18-20 years of their life babysitting this child". To each, his own.

But from what I have seen, in the balance, the number of those who harbour the desire to have a family of their own is a lot higher. Any statistic on this matter can be debated heavily, but one thing that no one can ignore is the growth and increasing population of maternity services and fertility clinics. Research reports suggest that the Indian IVF market alone is growing at 15% per annum and will touch USD 1.5 billion by 2026. This trend proves one simple fact - having babies isn't going out of fashion any time soon.

What has changed, however, is that people are no longer in a hurry to have kids. Women are opting to get a higher education, sometimes well into their late 20s, and want to build the foundation of their career before they get tied down by marital bonds or the responsibility of children. I, myself, for example, finished CA at 23 and didn't start seriously considering marriage until 26. And that was a decade ago. That trend has only progressed faster.

Better education and improved medical care facilities have increased the lifespans of people, further bolstering the trend of late parenting. The life expectancy of an average Indian today is around 68 years, as against 61 years 2 decades ago. In Japan, that number is as high as 84, while in the United States of America, the average life expectancy is 76 years. It basically means that people have longer to plan families. The meaning of the biological clock for you is different from that of your parents.

The quintessential urban couple looking to start a family averages between 27 and 35 years of age. I was 30 when I had my first child, and my husband was 32. Like most people in our friend and professional circles, we each have multiple degrees and had been fending for ourselves for almost 10 years by the time we had our first child. This trend is increasingly representative of the tier-II and tier-III cities.

The assumption would then be that such couples would have their finances well in place before having a baby. But that's not the case with everyone. The early years of a person's professional life don't always see much in terms of saving or future building. For some, it's because of the carelessness of youth and a lack of responsibility. For others, there are education loans being paid off or some other financial burden that needs to be addressed. For the more fortunate ones, there's the whole YOLO (You Only Live Once) mindset.

I had a bunch of things I wanted to do before I got married, and then my husband and I had a set of things we thought we wanted to do together before we had children. Backpacking vacations, adventurous pursuits like skydiving, scuba diving certifications, a smart home, and a better car were a few that we had. These things definitely cost a lot of money. So, although we were making a decent living, we didn't actually save as much as we could have in those years.

There's a focus on the fulfilment of hitherto unheard-of goals like exotic foreign travel, sabbaticals between job changes, and the desire for further education. Many couples feel they want to save up enough money and reach a certain level in their profession before they have a child or children. This does sound sensible, doesn't it? But achieving these goals, material or otherwise, comes at a cost price. And that's what this book is about. The price one must pay to have a baby. The first cost is the most irreplaceable resource we each have – time.

You need to give time to work, to your hobbies or interests, to your family, your responsibilities, and your life. But dedicating those years to these other things can lead to problems you didn't seriously think about.

For women especially, as much as I hate to admit it, the biological clock is always running. You may not know it, but a woman is actually born with all the eggs she will ever have in her ovaries. So once a girl starts getting her period, she is essentially already running the race against time involuntarily. Yeah, the joke's on us. Through this book, I want to draw not only on my own experience in planning a family but will also draw upon the expertise of some of the best-known names in gynaecology and obstetrics in India to help wannabe parents plan better the process of parenthood.

While I was carrying my youngest child, I did a lot of soul-searching. I forced myself to acknowledge many things that I hadn't in my earlier pregnancies. I had gone through so many difficulties during each one, not just physical and emotional but also logistical and practical; so much uncertainty as a mother-to-be and even as a person; so much pain and fear; innumerable moments of inexplicable despair and terribly sharp self-judgement. And, somehow, despite the multitude of people around me, despite my loving and caring partner's unerring presence, I had felt alone. I had battled without voicing out my fears, and I had borne without the courage to voice what I felt.

One of the biggest mistakes I made was not to voice these things properly to my husband. Maybe I didn't know better, maybe I didn't know how. Whatever the reason, in hindsight, it was a mistake. I should've shared my burden with him, and I should've asked him to share his. It was a mistake we both made. And I can't lie by saying that only I suffered. He went through his share of problems, uncertainties, and fears. While it was a beautiful time in our lives, something today we speak of fondly and smile about, it was also difficult. Maybe sharing would've made things better then…

Ideally, the elders and seniors in our lives should've told us about these things. They should've had the prescience to forewarn us about the rollercoaster this journey of becoming a parent is. Surely, they too, had gone through these feelings and problems, even if in different measures? Surely, they knew how difficult it could all be on a particular day? Then, why had no one shared any of these things with us? Why had no one told us the raw truth about trying to have a baby? Why had no one told us what would really go into the whole process? Or how it would, at times, tear my being apart and make me cry bitter tears? Or that the process would make him question his decisions and his self-confidence? No one helped us understand that it's not like what they show in the movies.

No one told my husband that he would need to be prepared for meltdowns, disappointment, and feelings of inadequacy. No one told him that he would have to go through my pain as badly as I did. I didn't even know that he would be going through problems of his own because this was as much his journey as it was mine.

Because I really wish someone had told us all of this, I'm doing it. I'm going to share with you what trying to become a parent is really about. The process of trying to have a baby is really trying. You might go through months upon months of frustration, and even if you conceive quickly, it won't be an easy ride.

When I tell you all of these things, I'm not on a mission to stop you from fulfilling your dream of becoming a parent. My intention is to prepare you for this ride, with its bumps, potholes, detours, and surprises. It is a beautiful, rewarding, and priceless journey that you intend to embark on. Therefore, it's only befitting that you prepare in every possible way for it.

I only hope that for every person who reads this book, there will be one person less who will struggle the way I did; maybe something in this book will make someone's journey easier and, perhaps, more joyful. Maybe you will find an informed, non-judgmental, unwavering companion in a really important part of your life! One that will make the price you pay for having your baby totally worth it!

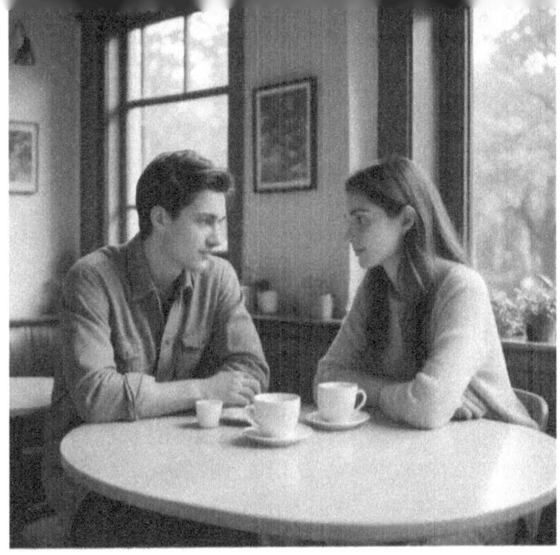

Chapter 1

COMMUNICATION AND CONSENT

Siddharth and Charmi met at a mutual friend's place while she was completing her graduation, and he was working for a Mumbai-based construction company. Siddharth came from a tier-II city business family, and Charmi was the daughter of a reasonably affluent stockbroker. It wasn't love at first sight, but fall in love they did eventually. When Siddharth popped the big question after 5 years of dating, it wasn't an immediate yes from her. The concerns were about having to leave her beloved city to move to a smaller place and around her career. He wasn't sure his parents would be too thrilled about their bahu going out for a job. That he wanted children early while she wanted to study further didn't help matters. No, things didn't work out eventually.

Siddharth and Charmi's story is fairly common. For most people, the search for a partner is a long-drawn and difficult process. They meet different people, figure out whether or not they are going to get along, and eventually, something clicks with someone. While this discovery process for the perfect partner is long enough, the journey from getting into the relationship to taking it to the next level is the longer one for a lot of people. Not everyone feels they can spend the rest of their lives with someone they really like for now.

Some relationships don't work out because of compatibility issues. Some don't work because of external factors like distance and family. Some fall apart because both don't want the same thing. At the same time, people end up getting married for a lot of reasons other than eternal love. Fear of loneliness, parental pressure, and economic reasons could be anything. Even in the 21st century, people are marrying someone their birth date or parents said they were compatible with, as Siddharth did a couple of years later. Don't get me wrong; there's no judgement here; I'm one of them. However, the idea is that marriage has a lot to do with convenience rather than happiness in our world. Whatever the reason for being together, communication is key.

I had a stereotypical Indian arranged marriage. A shock for most of my friends who were used to the girl with this independent, 'devil may care' attitude. But I had always maintained one thing – if both my parents and my brother liked a guy, I would gladly marry him. Simply because that's the kind of equation I had with them – one of immense love and trust where I knew they would want nothing but the best for me. That's how I met my husband and the father of my children. One day, we were strangers, 2 days later, we were engaged, and 2 months later, we were married.

For people who are like me and are married to someone they don't know very well (assuming that anyone knows anybody else well at all!), it's critical that you both first spend time getting to know each other. The idea of living with a stranger seems rather strange until you're one of those who took the irrational leap of faith based on the rational laid out for you by someone else. Whatever the case, before actually having a family together, you're going to need to figure out each other. Fundamentally, you need to be able to do 3 things before you make the call:

✳ Get to know each other.

✳ Settle into a new ecosystem, whether with an extended family or by yourselves.

✳ Ensure you have your professional life on track before you can undergo more changes.

Even when you're married to someone you dated, there are questions that need to be answered and compatibility issues that need to be worked on once you both actually start living together. This is not easy to accomplish, and while you're unlikely to have walked down the aisle without establishing some amount of compatibility, it is important to iron out any major issues before actually starting a family. Never take anything for granted, especially because many people who are often coaxed into an arranged marriage by their families may not really be ready for the next step in their new lives.

Consent is really crucial for both partners because it is truly a monumental decision and something that will affect both of you in every aspect of your life. If the clarity that both want the same thing, including children, is not there, then it becomes difficult to make the relationship work. Raising a child is a loooooooootttttttt of work. You don't want to have to go it alone as far as possible.

You can make an informed decision only if you truly appreciate what it really means to have a baby. Unless both of you know exactly what it means and how it would impact *the life you want to have together*, it would be a rash decision. The changes a child will cause in your life – I mean, you won't even recognise it as your own. What does having a kid really imply? For starters:

✳ Turning your lives upside down in every possible way.

✳ This is for a person who wouldn't exist if you chose not to bring her into your life.

* Providing for this person financially, physically, and emotionally in every living moment and

* Putting the needs of someone else before your own.

Are you both sure you really want to be parents? If you are and your partner isn't, please talk and sort it out. It could be that while you are sure, your partner is either unsure for a variety of reasons or totally against it. It's important to actually have the conversation before you start trying to get pregnant. You also don't want to ruin your relationship because you didn't give adequate importance to your partner's consent.

Communicating about this matter is not just about getting a yes or no answer. Letting your partner know what you want and asking them what they want is paramount. It's as much about respect as anything else. You wouldn't want your partner to force their wishes onto you, and therefore, you shouldn't be doing this to them.

Do everything you can to ensure clear communication on this matter because once you've committed to parenthood, there's no looking back. No 'Ctrl-Z' on this one. Love and commitment are 2 different things. Don't confuse readiness to be with you for readiness to be a parent.

If you both don't agree on the idea of parenting, you might have to evaluate the basic premise of the relationship. I know most couples talk about whether they'd like to have a family together or not at some point. It's a question that can be the deal-breaker when dating someone and deciding whether or not the relationship should be taken forward. If your desire to have a child is going to come in the way of your partner's aspirations, you might have to consider the alternatives seriously. Because, sometimes, 3 is a crowd.

At this point, I want you to ask yourselves a few questions:

What kind of relationship is yours? Is it the kind where a new idea is welcomed and evaluated or one where changes are avoided?

Is your foundation strong? What really holds the both of you together?

Will your equation change if there is a baby? Will it be able to survive the insecurities a child might cause?

Do you truly believe that you both have what it takes to build a family unit together? Are you both capable of sharing responsibility and making adjustments as and when the need arises?

If most of these are answered with a yes, there is clearly a green flag. An old friend of mine from my CA days is married to a girl he met through a professional matchmaking service. They're both highly intelligent, intellectual people. They had a strong marriage for 4 years before the question of children was discussed. She wasn't sure earlier, and he was clear that they would have children only if she really wanted them. For him, it wasn't a personal need or the opposite for having a kid. It was just not that important to him. When she came clean and discussed the topic with him, he supported her wish and went through with the idea. They have a son now, and my friend is a fantastic, doting father.

The good thing for them was that he let her decide and assured her that either way, he would support her. There was no resistance or preference from his side, but that didn't mean that it would not be his decision as well. He participated in the decision and followed through on it. All in, no second thoughts. That kind of clarity can be hard to find, but it's worth looking for.

Maybe one of you is more dominant in the relationship? Being dominant doesn't mean being pushy or bossy. It could mean that what one person usually prefers usually goes. It could be because one partner appreciates the intelligence and thought process of the other, or it could be because your partner would rather avoid a fight. In my case, neither of us is really dominant, but at times when we don't necessarily agree on a matter, one goes along sometimes because of the first reason and sometimes the second. If you are the dominant one, then you don't want to dump this onto your partner. It is going to be an enduring change in your lives. Please ask how your better half feels about it: is he/she up to being a parent? Does he feel he wants it, but maybe not right away?

Where the relationship is solid, and one partner is confident that it will hold through the pressures of a kid, then it's worth trying to bring your partner on the same page. A small test check could be trying to have a pet.

A college friend of mine and his wife met at a Metallica concert. Their bond over music turned into the symphony of life. Also, they both initially didn't want kids. I wasn't surprised because I never thought he was the father type. They got a Labrador and were really happy having a four-legged baby. Eight years later, they found out that they were pregnant and decided to go through with the pregnancy. He once told me that having the dog had given them a taste of consistent responsibility which neither of them had been used to. It made the possibility of having a baby worth considering.

I also feel you shouldn't let something like this become a filter between the both of you. Make it a cause for thought instead – by drawing parallels between the kind of relationship that either of you shares with your parents or by considering the potential for a "little me" in your lives. Talk about why you want the baby and leave room for why not to have one. If you can't find common ground now, most likely, it will become an insurmountable rift between you in the future. Then again, if you know that your partner didn't share a great relationship with his or her folks, it doesn't mean that you can't have a beautiful one with your own kids.

If your partner feels positive about the whole thing but feels the time is not right now, it's fine. You can evaluate the 'when' a little later. You will need to do a lot of planning, and that planning process will give both of you enough time to sort things in your mind as well. If your partner is not positive about it, then you have to also understand why. Here's a list of questions you may want to ask your partner to understand where the roadblock is:

✳   Is the thought of being a parent alien?

✳   Where is the roadblock in the thought process?

✳   Is it a question of the responsibility being too much?

✳   Is it the fear of losing their freedom?

✳   Maybe they don't know how they will cope with the financial responsibility.

✳   Maybe he/she is scared the baby will displace him/her in your life.

✳   Is there something in their past that makes them not want to be tied down?

✳   Maybe they just don't know how they will fare as a parent.

A person's insecurity can have a lot more to do with themselves than with those around them. As a life partner, it becomes your responsibility to first share in that trauma and help deal with it before you propose to further complicate your partner's life. So don't take this lightly. You may need to gain the confidence of your partner in ways you never thought you would need to. It means getting to know your partner more holistically and focusing on their needs over yours.

A designer friend married her college sweetheart. They're amazing together, but they're both very laid-back, indecisive people. She's the sort who can never say no to anyone, no matter what. And he's the sort who can't say yes to anything you ask him; he's always 'thinking it over.' They married at 24, straight out of design school, but couldn't decide on having a baby even after 12 years of marriage. I'd keep asking her if they'd spoken about it, and she would keep telling me, "Sourabh's not said yes; he's not said no." It was really getting to her.

The problem was that although both were great designers, neither was doing very well professionally, and they weren't sure how they would afford the baby. He was having a hard time saying no outright Are You Ready For Your Baby, Yet?because he didn't want to hurt her. She really longed for one and couldn't understand why he wasn't agreeing. It wasn't until her sister pushed them into having a face-off on the subject that he admitted his fears about financial instability. He had a fair point. They were sort of living paycheck to paycheck. The fear of not being able to provide the kind of life they would want for the child was so great that eventually, she dropped the idea. I know, now as a friend, that the decision hasn't been easy for them, and she's still coming to terms with it, but that's where things are.

The point is basically this: You could think of a child as an ambitious, high-risk, high-return joint project that 2 people decide to embark upon. Ambitious because you are looking at moving your relationship to the ultimate level of commitment – starting a family together. High-risk because not only life after the baby eventually, but even the pregnancy is fraught with all kinds of possibilities. High-return because the pay-off is priceless – pure, unadulterated love. But just like you wouldn't get into a joint venture with someone without their full, explicit consent, you don't want to get onto the parenting juggernaut without your partner's explicit acceptance of the idea.

One rule, however, doesn't apply to all. A lot of people who aren't the confrontational sort choose to drop subtle hints. They share their feelings of longing while claiming to be on the fence about the baby. They profess complete focus on their partner but allow for the feeling of something being incomplete. What this does is it tells them that he/she is most important and that nothing is complete if they don't share the joy in it. Let your partner know in subtle ways what a baby would add to your life and build on the topic. Let them start living your dream, one snooze at a time. As Daniel Kahnemann says in his fantastic book, "Thinking, Fast And Slow," priming is a critical influence on one's thought process. You might want to try it.

If your parents matter in the equation and have been harping about when they'll hear "the good news," then the topic becomes easier to deal with. Let them take the lead in pushing for the decision. You get to play good cop and still get what you want. At the same time, don't let it sound like something you're doing only for the parents. Eventually, it's your life and your responsibility. So let it still be a call the 2 of you are making for yourselves. The parents are a good excuse to push the discussion, that's all.

However, be mindful that bringing up sensitive topics too often can end up hurting the relationship. Let it come from him/her once in a while. All it sometimes takes is you looking longingly at the adorable kid in the newspaper ad or you accidentally leaving your phone unlocked and the browser on some website for nursery furniture! One could say this is overkill, but priming is a better way to look at it.

Give it time. Go slow and steady. It's better that it be a decision that both of you made together. Once your partner comes around and agrees that, yes, both of you should start a family, you can feel more confident in your decision as well. Don't let any of the negativity get to you. I know a lot of the questions I've raised can sound daunting, but the most difficult questions in life are often the most important ones. Answering them now rather than later will give you more confidence in your decision and make your life easier in the long run.

So yes, work on getting those answers. They will make a difference. After all, as C.S. Lewis said, "Children are not a distraction from more important work. They are the most importantly work."

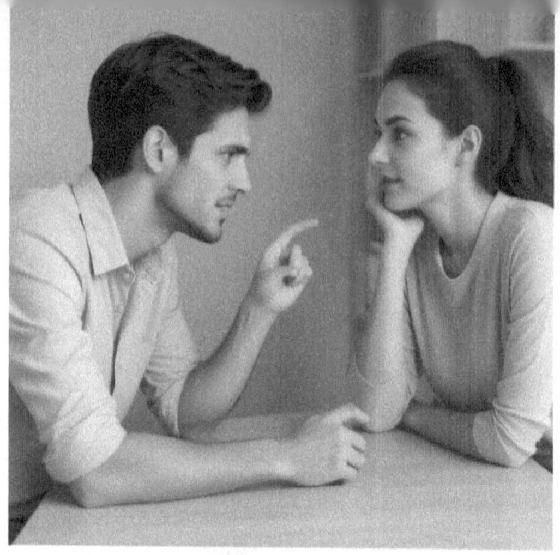

Chapter 2

TIMING

Vishal met his wife, Mini, when they were both in twelfth grade. They secretly dated for the next 4 years before he wanted to move to Bangalore to complete his articleship for CA. They told their parents about each other, and the ultimatum from Mini's family was very clear – either you guys get married, or we'll start looking for a suitable match for her. A conservative Brahmin family, a graduate girl, and all that. They took the plunge and got married when they were barely 22 years old. But the baby didn't happen until almost 10 years later. Not only did he need to find his feet and become independent, but she also wanted to study further; her parents were less supportive of this than her husband was. She went on to get into the Indian Institute of Science and did her post-graduation in Materials Science. Even then, they wanted to move to the US because her options for employment in India were seemingly limited. So, they did. They are now settled happily with their twin boys in Arizona.

Then again, there's the story of my cousin, Preeti. Preeti was our family's beauty queen. The prettiest of all of us cousin sisters and definitely the most pampered. She barely got through graduation. My aunt had started boy-hunting for her even before Preeti had written her B.Com. Final exams. Given how pretty she was and apparently docile, there was no shortage of rishtas for her. But, this perfect bahu material girl had one clear condition – no babies for at least 3 years after marriage. That didn't go down too well with most potential in-laws because they felt that if a girl had such conditions before marriage, you could ostensibly gauge what kind of tantrums she might throw afterwards! This was a rather unfair and insensible assessment of a girl who knew exactly what she wanted out of life. Having seen her mother and older sister go through the same cycle, Preeti was amply clear that since any which way she would have to get into the inevitable grind of marriage-kids-responsibilities, she might as well have a chance to live her life. Hence, the condition.

Now, a lot of us know at some point in life whether or not we have the parenting gene. I knew that pretty early, actually. It was something that was always going to be a big part of who I am. But that didn't mean I was ready to bite the proverbial bullet straight after marriage. While having the clarity that yes, both of you want a family together is great, figuring out the right time of your life to have that family can be complicated. And whether that time is now or not, well, difficult to tell without a lot of thought. While you may or may not have control over when you get married, what you should try to plan better is WHEN you start trying for a baby.

See, our families are no longer the way our parents' or grandparents' were. There are no predefined gender roles, and there is no single breadwinner. Most families these days are multi-income households. So, even the question of when the family is ready for a baby is not dependent on one person. It is as important for the mother to be ready for it as it used to be in the days of yore for the father. Like in the case of Vishal and Mini, although Vishal was reasonably settled in his career and life by 28, Mini was unhappy with the opportunities she got in her field in India and wanted to be sorted in that before she committed herself to motherhood. So, they took a few more years not only to relocate to a different country but also to establish their lives there.

This question of timing is also not just dependent on career or life goals. A lot of people get into parenting believing that their life will come to a standstill, like my cousin. That may not happen to everyone, but having a child is a game-changer in the sense that it makes it impossible to make spontaneous decisions. Therefore, even if you don't have a major checklist to tick off before you get rolling, it is worth being all set in your mind for the ensuing journey. Parenthood is not the end of life, but certainly of life as you know it. Lifestyle and mindset modifications will be many and drastic.

The idea of timing is relevant for another very important difference in our times compared to our parents. To give you context, let me tell you a story about the day I was born. My mother had gone for a routine check-up to her gynaec, and the doctor told her that there seemed to be something wrong with my heartbeat. She would have to be operated on immediately. At that point, mom was around 8 months pregnant and at least 2 weeks ahead of the delivery date. My aunt (dad's older brother's wife) was with mom for the check-up, and she called a couple of relatives who were living in the area to inform them of the surgery. My dad was out for work and didn't know of my birth until late that night. These were the times when landlines were not that common, even before cell phones. He came home to find out that he was father to a -7pound baby girl!

Can you imagine being in my mom or dad's place? Having the baby without adequate notice? Or the father not being around at the time of the kid's birth? None of us living in the 21st century can actually dream of being such 'careless,' 'disinterested' or 'uninvolved' parents. My parents were none of these; they were just regular 20th-century first-time parents belonging to the generation we now call baby boomers!

Nowadays, both parents want to be there for the minutest milestone of the child – the first sound, the first word, the first crawl, and the first step! Missing your child's birth is unthinkable. We want to be there for all of this, right? But only when we are "ready" for the baby.

This readiness is not simply a state of mind. It is the net result of a number of factors. These factors are emotional, financial, and logistical. The first among those is, of course, your relationship status. Either you are with someone with whom you would like to plan a family, and you have both reached a mutual decision on wanting to start one, or you are one of those people who want to pursue parenthood on your own. Either way, you should've established that you want to do it. There is no right or wrong, and you really need to know what you are doing, whether in partnership or solo.

My husband and I, in the 45 minutes that we spoke before we were engaged to each other, discussed the topic of kids. We were both sure we wanted them, but like my cousin, I don't think I was ready for kids immediately after marriage. The maternity gene was there, alright, but it needed time to mature! My husband had been around babies all his life, but I hadn't been within a mile of one in the family for nearly 20 years. He was alright with that. He acknowledged that I needed time to get to know him, settle down in a whole new ecosystem, and restructure my professional life. I'm glad we discussed all of this because even in hindsight, I know I would not have been able to deal with the baby the way I eventually did before all of this was sorted. Similarly, your *readiness* could be linked to any kind of factors, and unless you identify them, you won't know how to address them or when you will be as ready as you can ever be!

I'm just wondering, have you thought of your life in terms of a timetable? It's something we all do at one point in life or another. It goes like this: finish education by Year **M**, reach a certain level of salary or savings by Year **N**, be married or in a serious relationship by Year **O**, and then, of course, that magical age, Year **P**, by which you should become pregnant! While many of these things happen on autopilot because of the way our educational system is structured, in the latter part of our lives, achieving the milestones of this timetable per schedule can be very difficult. Sometimes the best of plans don't work out. But, having a plan is important because it gives you something to work towards and also some semblance of control over your life. That sense of control may be misplaced (as I've discovered more often than not), but just the planning process can be comforting at the very least!

These timetables are not always our own doing. For people who live among a lot of relatives and are from a more traditional mindset, there's always pressure to move into the next stage of life. If you're studying, people ask about when you'll become financially independent. Once you are financially independent, they ask about marriage. And from the day after your marriage, the questions about when you're going to have a kid start. People living away from all this drama have it easier, but the timetable of life still persists. The pressure is often self-induced or just laid on by well-meaning family and friends.

Don't let the questions get to you. This life is yours, and so should the decisions be. Unless you are confident that the time has come for you to embark on such a wonderful yet difficult journey, you would be doing a great disservice to yourself by hopping onto the parenting rollercoaster. The state of readiness that you need to reach to do so will come after you have done the things that come most naturally to you – whether it is becoming professionally successful, whether it is taking care of certain family commitments or whether it is fulfilling non-obligatory personal desires.

You've invested so much of your life in your career and education. Therefore, it's only natural that you would have set the achievement of certain career benchmarks or goals as a parameter before moving on to other things in life. What you may want to do is to figure out what that benchmark is for both of you. First, discuss what these goals are and how long realistically you need to achieve these. See what the timelines for these goals look like and how they compare with the biological clock you guys are or will be up against. Unless you assess that, you won't know how long it's going to be before you can seriously plan a baby.

A friendly piece of advice: beware of over-optimism. Don't try to tell yourself you can achieve in 3 years what others take 6 years to do. You're setting this as a turning point or a pivot in your life. It is better to be realistic about it.

At the same time, talk to your friends or peers and understand what all of them are thinking in this context. Some points you may want to discuss with them are:

* Are your peers thinking about kids?
* How long do they want to wait before they have a kid?
* How financially prepared are they?
* How do your close friends perceive you?
* Do they see you as someone who could graduate into being a parent soon?
* How long do they feel you should wait before you start trying for a baby?

Talking to people who are a little ahead of you in terms of age and experience is also as beneficial as talking to your like-age friends and peers. Asking slightly older friends about how long they took to plan their kid, what kind of thoughts went on in their mind before they did it, and how they knew they were finally ready to take the plunge will all help you make up your mind as well. Talk to them about their careers and how they positioned themselves before you start planning.

I can't stress how important it is to sort out your careers; after all, raising a child these days isn't cheap. The cost of pregnancy and then delivery put together is easily as much as someone's annual savings or maybe even their income for a year. Post-delivery, there will be a number of fixed and variable costs. While some of these costs will taper off by the time the child is 2, like monthly vaccinations, others will be replaced by the cost of education. So, you have to be financially sound in order to provide comfortably for yourself and your family.

Money is certainly a huge consideration, but is your own happiness and sense of fulfilment not equally paramount? You wouldn't want to be in a position where either you or your partner is having to forego a foreign posting or a job change because you're having a baby. At the same time, the parent who is going to bear the greater burden of parenting shouldn't end up feeling like he/she drew the short straw. The timing is about all of these things. If you get the timing right, it won't feel like a sacrifice or a mistake. If the timing is wrong, it could end up dampening your joy and sense of fulfilment in other spheres of life.

When I talk about the greater burden of parenting, I don't necessarily mean the biological mother. Many modern fathers are not averse to taking up less demanding job profiles or even career breaks to take care of their children because their wives/husbands are unable or undesirous to do so. How they deal with any stigma of doing it is another matter. But it's definitely a choice these days, and fewer people are likely to judge them than before. And make no mistake, 2 people running behind big careers without adequate support don't make for an ideal family.

A lady I know from my prenatal classes quit her consulting career to become a professional baker. It was a passion she had harboured all her life. After her daughter turned 1, she applied for a baking course in a different city and was accepted. However, within a few days of receiving her acceptance letter, she found out she was expecting her second baby. This threw her into turmoil. She and her husband had originally planned on having only 1 child. She wasn't sure she could go through with this because her course started in 6 months. It was a tough decision, but eventually, her husband promised to take care of the younger one as soon as the baby was weaned off so that she could take up the course but a year later. He came good on his word. She did complete the course. Now, she runs her niche baking studio from an apartment in suburban Mumbai, with one room turned into a nursery for her kids.

It's usually also a good idea to understand how the couple stacks up on the age metric. If you're on the wrong side of 30, while it's not late at all to have the first child, you might have a slightly harder time doing it than someone 5 years younger. Whatever your age, it might not be a bad idea to get some help to ensure that you have as good a chance as any of having kids of your own.

This would include seeking medical advice and learning about the options available for freezing your sperm and eggs. If you are quite young and know that having children is a definite possibility in the future, but you're not sure when it will happen, it makes sense to freeze your eggs/sperm early on. It's not an easy process because it will require the egg donor to take some medication and many hormonal injections to increase the production of eggs. However, it will save her tons of angst and any potential disappointment if she does end up opting for late pregnancy. It's not very expensive and will also be extremely helpful if IVF is ever needed. If you know that you're already in your late 20s or early to mid30-s and need to wait a few more years before having a baby, freezing your eggs or sperm could be a great idea insofar as the surety of having a biological child is needed.

Expert Speak
Freezing of Eggs & Sperm

Nowadays, an occasional lady comes in and inquiries about egg freezing. What is the freezing of gametes? Gametes is the scientific word for eggs or oocytes and sperms. Normally, males ejaculate millions of sperms in a single ejaculate. On the other hand, a woman's ovary releases only one oocyte or egg in any given month. Occasionally, more than one egg gets released and if both get fertilised, a twin pregnancy results.

As a woman ages, her ovarian reserve reduces so that as she becomes older, she may not ovulate in each month, or even if she ovulates, the oocytes may not be as healthy as those of a younger woman. Thus, a woman's fertility declines with age. On the other hand, the male sperm count does not deteriorate as significantly with age. Unless the male undergoes some major treatment that affects his overall physical fitness, his fertility is unlikely to be significantly affected. This applies even more to women as their bodies will also be affected by any major surgery or prolonged treatment. In such circumstances, when the individual is young and desirous of preserving fertility, doctors may advise cryopreservation or freezing of gametes.

In men, it's a relatively simple procedure. The man is asked to give a semen sample by masturbation, and the semen sample is then frozen for retrieval and thawing at a later date. The issue is more complex in women. Women need to be hyper-stimulated with hormones so as to let their ovaries produce multiple eggs at one time. The eggs or oocytes have then to be retrieved by needle aspiration under the guidance of sonography in a procedure that is performed in an operation theatre. The retrieved oocytes are then frozen for future use. This is a much more complicated and expensive procedure as compared to the process in males.

Thus, though freezing of eggs and sperms in the modern world is feasible, perhaps it is best reserved for medical reasons or for the occasional woman who is completely occupied with either her education, her profession or some other priority and chooses to undertake the rather arduous process of harvesting and freezing her oocytes to ensure her capability to reproduce in the future.

The hazards of modern life and the toll they cause place great stress on one's body. Poor lifestyles are the single biggest contributors to the coffers of fertility clinics. There's very little wrong with us when we're born; it's what we do to ourselves thereafter that causes the problems! That's why I feel each person needs to be more aware of their own body and how they are mistreating it. PCOS, irregular menstrual cycles, and low sperm counts are all often the result of man-made habits. If you can put as much effort into taking care of your mental and physical well-being as you do with your professional well-being, you will realise later that it is worth the investment.

I've had PCOS since my teens. Years of long nights studying and then pulling all-nighters in the office meant that I didn't pay much attention to my health. Honestly, I didn't have the time to do much about it either. It wasn't until after I quit my corporate job that I got back to working on my fitness. These days, people are smarter about it. There's greater awareness (or so I hope) and generally, people do appreciate the long-term benefits of attending to their fitness as well. But it would be good for you to invest at least half an hour a day in some form of exercise and eat more consciously. You don't want to be found wanting physically during crunch times.

Expert Speak

Today, practically every day, a woman will walk into the clinic, telling you she has PCOD (D stands for disease) or PCOS. When you ask her what her complaints or issues are, she will give a slightly exasperated look, wondering whether you are daft and reiterate, "Doc, I told you that I have PCOS." And you patiently ask once again, "Can you tell me what exactly is bothering you?"

"Polycystic ovaries" is an appearance of the ovaries on ultrasound where the ovaries appear bulky and plump and have a string of tiny pearl-like cysts forming a necklace around the edge of the ovaries. These cysts are not actually cysts but are eggs or follicles that have partially developed, but then the development did not progress, and the eggs did not get released.

During a woman's reproductive life, that is the time between menarche and menopause, the ovaries invariably release one egg every month. In ladies with PCO, there is a hormonal imbalance, which may lead to anovulation or the absence of egg release. However, it should be remembered that just having a polycystic appearance on ultrasound does not necessarily mean that ovulation is absent.

If there is anovulation, the lady may present either with irregular periods or infertility. The periods may be delayed, or the flow may be scanty, or there may be excessive bleeding after a prolonged period of absent menses. PCO is also known to be associated with other conditions, such as insulin resistance, where the body does not respond to insulin's action. There may be diabetes and weight gain. Some ladies have extraordinarily excessive weight gain, while others may remain slim. Excess and abnormal distribution of hair may be seen. Acne and darkened pigmentation at the nape of the neck and elbows are also often present. Sometimes, cholesterol and triglycerides are unfavourably raised.

The management of PCOD depends on what the patient is complaining about. Just because the ovaries appear polycystic on sonography does not mean that the woman needs treatment. Increasing one's activity level with daily brisk walks for approximately 30-45 minutes can break the steady state of anovulation and may sometimes be all that is needed. If the lady wants to conceive, she can be helped with medications that help to get the egg ready. If she does not wish to have a baby, keeping her on oral contraceptive pills helps to regulate the menstrual cycle as well as correct the abnormal hormone profile. Sometimes, only progesterone medications are used to regulate the cycle. If there is an excess of male hormone secretion, an occasional woman will benefit from the use of anti-androgen medicines. A woman with insulin resistance will benefit from the use of the anti-diabetic medication called metformin.

Thus, the management of a woman with polycystic ovaries will depend on her needs.

People often have many other goals which are not strictly related to their careers. These could be something related to their personal lives or their families. Planning is important in order to even start checking these things off your to-do list, especially if they're things you would ideally want to be done with before your personal responsibilities and financial obligations grow in the aftermath of pregnancy.

You might need to save more money than before for the things that are really important to you. You may also need to dedicate more time to doing these things that you feel you may not get an opportunity to do later in life. Along with finding time to keep yourself fit, both physically and mentally, it is also important to take care of things that make a difference to your emotional well-being. Whether it's sending your parents on an all-expenses-paid holiday, finishing an executive MBA, or making sure your younger sibling is married, it will all need time, money, and effort. The more you procrastinate, the harder it'll become for you to step back from a fast-paced life when you decide to plan your family. Therefore, factor in all kinds of goals that could end up on your list of regrets in 25 years if not addressed now.

The factors you should jot down and work on would largely fall into 5 buckets:

1. Physical readiness.
2. Ability to mentally commit to a baby.
3. Financial stability.
4. Fulfilling any major personal goals or achieving personal milestones that might be hindered by small child responsibilities.
5. Any family-related to-dos that would prevent you from focusing on your own and the child's health if not addressed earlier.
6. Anything related to the long-term goals you set for yourself, which you must start servicing before you start working on your family planning.

The flip side to all of this is, you can never really be ready enough. There is always going to be fear and uncertainty. For a lot of people, I know that the uncertainty comes from the financial aspect and from the fear of commitment. If your partner is dealing with either of these, you may or may not be able to fully convince them about being ready enough. You might have to just convince them that out of 6 things, you guys are good on 4 and it's time to move on. If that's the case, the discussion will have to be managed very carefully. You don't want to make it look like the baby was your decision alone. It can cause a lot of undue blame-dumping in the future.

Try using the list of headings I've suggested above and see how you guys fare on each of them. Sometimes, you may not be doing very well in even 4 of them, but you might still feel like the time is right. That's fine. Ultimately, if you feel ready and if this is what you want and you want it now,

Then there's no reason to look back or to hesitate. No one can tell you how you're going to feel about it. So, although I would say try to make an informed decision, the final word should come from your heart.

At this point, I want to reiterate that having a baby is not the end of the world as you know it. True, life will change forever, and the freedom to pack bags at the drop of a hat will be curtailed for a while. But it doesn't mean that one can't have a career going forward or get further education. One of my greatest inspirations in this matter was a senior in the office back during my days at the Big4. This lady, married to a senior executive at the world's leading search engine, finished her CPA after having 3 kids. When my parents started asking me to get married, I would often discuss it with her, and she would always tell me that nothing needed to stop after marriage or with kids. She would say that so long as you are careful in choosing your partner and back yourself fully in doing what your heart wants, it can be made to happen. Then, I didn't really believe her, but today, more than 10 years of personal experience later, I do with all my heart.

Having a kid doesn't mean that to dream of trekking up Mount Everest or making an expedition to Antarctica is illogical. The time for all these things will come, BUT you don't know *how soon*. I once read somewhere that parenting is like using a GPS navigator that keeps recalculating every time you make a turn! That GPS starts pretty much the day the baby arrives, and you'll go off-road so many times that your appetite for adventure will take a hit. Believe me, I know what I'm talking about!

Please take a step back, introspect, and then choose a relaxed time to sit down with your partner to have a good discussion. It's worthwhile to draw up a timeline of when and how one can plan the process that will lead to you being prepared for parenthood. If it's that important to you or if, like me, it's inevitable in your life, surely you can invest that much time to think things through. There are no guarantees of anything in life, but surely, we can plan for the worst and hope for the best, always with a few calculated guesses!

PS: Attaching a sample checklist that could help you plan for this better.

Type of Goal	Particulars	Time required (in months)	Priority Score (out of 10)	Estimated Completion Date
Professional	Become a VP			
	Move abroad for work			
	Start a business			
Educational	PhD., MBA, Masters, etc			
Personal	Scuba diving course			
	Backpack through Europe			
	Etc			
Family	Younger brother's marriage			
	Buying mom a house			
	Sending dad on a foreign holiday			
	Replacing sister's car			
	Etc			
Physical	Lose weight			
	Control BP			
	Become fitter			
	Etc			
Financial	Buy a house			
	Buy a car			
	PIS ni shkal 01.sR			
	eerf tbed emoceB			
	ctE			

The items that have a priority score of less than 7 should be considered non-critical and items requiring more than 5 years if you're less than 30 or more than 3 years if you're more than 30, should be re-evaluated. If they're still critical, you might want to consider sperm/egg preservation for sure!

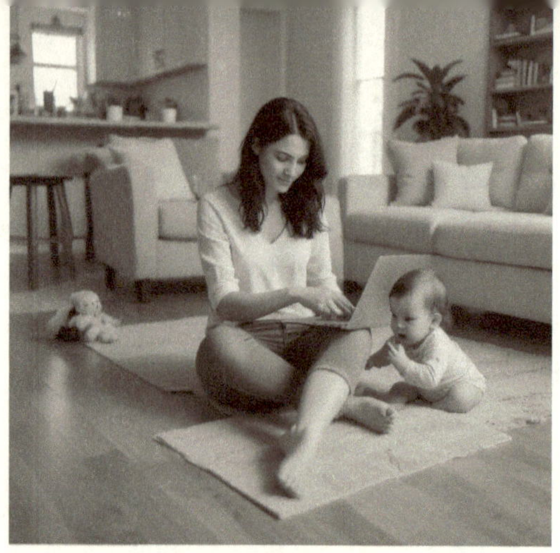

CARRYING YOUR CAREER ALONG WITH THE BABY

One of my seniors during my time at the Big4 was this amazing lady called Swati. Swati is one of the most technically sound and committed professionals you'll ever meet. She moved to Bangalore from Chennai after marriage and was always among the first to finish her assignments before tax audit season and always a top performer. She was so consistent and effective in her work that all of us could only wonder how she did it. When we suddenly found out that Swati, who had been in our office for almost 2 years, was 6 months pregnant, we were all blown away. She didn't tell us until her baby bump became obvious. No one who had seen this lady work like a maniac would have guessed in their wildest dreams that she was going through a pregnancy. The only additional support she had at home was her husband's aunt who lived with them. I asked her why she worked the way she did despite her pregnancy, and her answer really stumped me. She said, "Aarti, if I don't work the way

I'm used to working, I'll go crazy. My work keeps me sane." Even after her child was born, she took only 3 months of maternity leave and was back to working half days from the office immediately after.

Swati is no longer an exception in India. There are thousands of women out there, maybe lakhs, for whom their work is their connection to sanity. They have put a lot of effort into their careers, and it is a huge part of who they are. Giving up completely on something they've worked so hard to build is not an option. And although it demands a lot of physical exertion and immeasurable strength of mind, they derive comfort from the discipline that comes with sticking to their routine. It gives them a sense of normalcy when they no longer have control over how their bodies are going to behave or how their emotions are going to play out. However, this is not the case for everyone.

A lawyer called Lavanya I once met at a friend's place has an interesting story. Lavanya is a human rights lawyer, and like many in her profession, more often than not, she tends to get very consumed by the problems that her clients face. Right from problems related to child abuse and marital discord to police brutality and human rights violations, the things she lives through vicariously are painful. So naturally, this affects her state of mind as well. Her husband is also a lawyer, but a corporate one. His work is more neutral and not to mention, better paying. After being married for 10 years, they had adopted one baby girl but also wanted a biological child. Naturally, it was important that they figure out the "what, when, and how" before they got into the whole shebang of pregnancy. Because of the nature of Lavanya's work, her doctor advised her to take a short break because the stress was really working up her hormones and making it difficult for her to conceive. Although she had already frozen her eggs a few years ago, one cycle of IVF had failed because of the strain she was under.

Lavanya's story is not a case in point for women having to stop working in order to conceive. It's just testament to the impact of stress on our bodies. What happened to her was that she was physically unable to cope with the strain of her work. Cutting back on the amount of work she was taking on and being careful about the kind of cases she opted for helped manage her stress. This allowed her to find time to work on her mental health, which in turn had a great bearing on her physical wellness too. It didn't take very long for her to conceive eventually, and she did work through the rest of her pregnancy. The decision was to slow down, not stop.

Now that you have agreed on the fact that you want to start a family and the broad time horizon of when you want to have the baby, you need to understand how long before having the baby the process really starts. It's not quite like they show in the movies, you know. One fine day 2 people are married, and with a beautiful montage of passing seasons, there's a baby in the nursery! Many things affect your life, and if you are a working person, it is important to manage this critical aspect of your life before you get pregnant. You don't want to be in a position where it's either/or. If both your career and your baby are equally important, you need to plan towards balancing them as best as you can.

If you have figured out that you want to have the baby, let's say, 2 years from the date of your discussion and when you've finished reading this book, you'll need to start ticking off a checklist of necessary things. Whether you are like Swati or Lavanya, or either of their spouses, you will need to ensure you have put in place whatever support mechanisms you need to get through the pregnancy process. Multiple visits to the doctor, office work, household responsibilities, managing your own health and finances, are only a few of the things that you will be juggling. Do remember that finances are important in all of this, and not for one moment can you ignore the potential pitfalls of not having your monetary buffer in place.

Statistics say that in India, as many as %34-18 of women don't return to work post-pregnancy. For a country that at %27 already has the lowest rate of female participation in the workforce out of the BRICS countries, that's a very damning number. If you and I are to ensure we don't add to that statistic, our best ally is common sense and medium-term planning.

There are many questions you could start by asking yourself.

Is your current location capable of allowing you long-term growth in your career?

Is your current job relevant to your long-term plans?

Are you living in the city in which you want to raise your kids?

Do you want to be closer to your parents or support system?

Would you rather move to a less polluted or more well-connected city?

Are the educational opportunities in your current location commensurate with your expectations for your child?

If there are too many 'no' answers in this list, you may need to re-evaluate. A good amount of effort will go into planning your relocation. Relocation doesn't happen overnight, and getting to your desired destination may not be easy at all, so start early enough. Sometimes, even those 2 years aren't going to be enough.

Another former colleague of mine has a story relevant in this context. Although she's a couple of years younger than me, she got married just about a year after I did and moved to London thereafter. She's become pretty successful in her career, and she and her husband have bought a beautiful little house in the suburbs of London. But, they've had a difficult time trying to figure out whether or not to plan a kid. The reason for them is that they're both working, and since they've bought the house, they can't afford to lose one income. If they continue working and saving the way they are now, they'll be able to pay off their housing loan in another 3 years. But, the clock's ticking and they don't have support. Plus, daycare and nannies are really expensive in the UK. So, they don't know what to do!

Common enough. A lot of people move out of the country for work or studies and wait to move back home before starting a family or defer pregnancy for a really long time because of financial commitments. Childcare isn't easy, and getting paid help is extremely expensive in the developed world. So, often the decision to have a baby is deferred until the couple has moved back.

Does your current employer give you the option to relocate? You can check the company's website or you might be knowing in which other cities the company has offices. If the offices are there, talk to HR to understand what company policy around relocation is. If that's not a possibility, you might have to change your job in a couple of years, maybe sooner. Start doing your research on opportunities in your preferred location. Just in case your kind of jobs are harder to come by, you are potentially looking at a change in your profile as well. It could mean having to learn new skills, getting an additional qualification, or maybe even a complete change of nature of work. If your parents or older relatives have been telling you that having a baby has no impact on your career, in this one paragraph alone, I've given you the whole low-down on why that's bullshit.

You see how one decision impacts other things? It's not a baby that stops people from going back to work or building their careers; it is the circumstances that ruin careers. Nobody tells young people what factors they should take into consideration if they want to succeed in having a happy life. Lots of people give career advice, and after you have had the baby, loads of parenting advice. But IN BETWEEN THE 2, no one helps you plan. I'm not saying life will become perfect if you plan, but at least there will be fewer pitfalls and lesser loss in every sense – personal, professional, and physical. Why not hedge your risks while you still have the time, right?

This table can help you arrive at your decision better:

Parameter	Relevance (on a scale of 1 to 5)	Yes or No	Yes = 1, No = 0	Rating Score
	R		N	S = R*N
Are the educational institutions in your city good?				
Do you need to live with or close to your parents?				
If the answer to the previous question is yes, are you currently in the same city as your parents?				
Does your current employer allow for good maternity/ paternity benefits?				
Will you get good day care facilities (if you need them) in your location?				
Can you grow in your career/field in your current location?				

Note: While assigning relevance score, 5 is the most important and 1 is the least.

The maximum score you can arrive at using this table is 30. I would imagine that a score of less than 12 means that your current job/location needs a change. Anything more than that needs to be evaluated depending on your personal situations and inherent limitations. But at least, now you can have a better idea of how to decide if it's been difficult so far.

I got a score of 22 on this table. That's primarily because since I have my own set-up and live with family, there was no question of maternity/paternity benefits and the need for a daycare facility. Even if your score is on the lower side but changing jobs or location is not an option for you, you can evaluate things from a different angle.

We live in a world of increasing opportunities for working from home as well as flexible working hours. People with good experience and talent are able to negotiate better deals with potential or current employers and still continue their career trajectory without giving up on personal desires. You may have to show some flexibility yourself in terms of your role or the pay, but things are definitely better now than they were in the earlier part of the millennium. It's not a dead-end, and you can find your path through some smart navigation.

At the same time, many people who find that they can't cope with the strain of their corporate careers or are not able to get the deal they wanted, are creating their own niche. They are able to apply their passion and experience to creating profitable vocations. So many people are doing freelance work through online platforms that match potential customers with skilled professionals like writers, designers, coders, etc. Many are using their knowledge to start their own classes or small businesses. People are also pursuing their long-standing passion with the aid of social media. For instance, there's been a massive boom in the home-bakers, home-chef, and freelance artist segment; not to mention influencers and YouTube celebrities!

The possibilities unleashed by creative thinking combined with technology are endless. If you have the will, you will surely find the way!

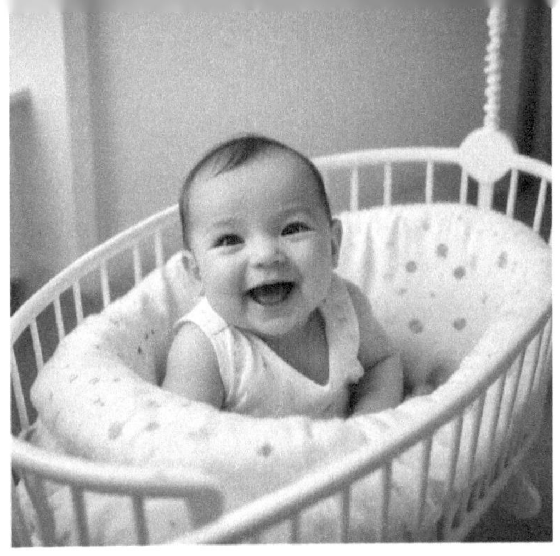

Chapter 4

SPACE FOR THE BABY

Kritika and Paul live in one of the prettiest sections of old Bandra. Their 60-year-old house was given to them by Paul's grandmother when they got married. They made a beautiful home of it and were preparing to welcome their first child into it. As the gifts during the baby shower poured in and they made a list of things they would need to have for the baby with the help of Kritika's prenatal classes and through online research, they realised that they had no room for either a large cot or a pram. As beautiful as their house was, it was a little cramped, and as Paul is a musician, the only spare bedroom was occupied by his mini-studio, full of musical instruments and paraphernalia.

It dampened their spirits for a few days. Until their friendly neighbour offered to let out his garage to them for Paul to set up his studio in. The money was a little tight, but they didn't have an option as Kritika's mother was also going to move in with them to help them look after the baby.

While everyone you meet will at some point ask you when you're planning for a baby or whether you're pregnant, nobody asks you whether you have done enough preparation in all the practical aspects of life before you think of having the baby. People can give you random advice on what kind of sexual positions will result in a guaranteed pregnancy or which foods are best consumed in order to conceive quickly, but no one actually tells you the magical formula to ensuring you've ticked the right boxes to make the arrival of the baby AND your life thereafter smooth.

Why is this so important, you ask? You may think that a roof over the head is good enough, and in an era where about one-fifth of the world's population lives in abject poverty, thinking in so much detail about what kind of house you live in is elitist. But that's not the case. The UK Government commissioned a study to understand the impact of bad housing conditions on the health, safety, ability to learn, and mental well-being of children. The study showed that children who grew up in bad housing conditions, had inadequate infrastructure, or lacked a positive and conducive environment, had more difficulty in learning during their formative years and eventually achieving economic well-being. This in turn affected their ability to succeed in life. This shows that comfortable housing and space are definitely important for the growth and well-being of children.

If you don't create the right conditions for your family to thrive in, you cannot question the pace of your family's overall growth. A home is not merely a place for sleeping; it provides a sense of belonging and symbolises our roots. Therefore, thoughtful consideration must precede your serious foray into family planning. Begin by creating the appropriate breeding ground (pun unintended!) for it.

Questions to consider

Is your home adequate for an extra person or 2? Where will the baby sleep? Is there space for a cot? Do your existing cupboards have enough room for the baby's clothes and accessories? Where will you store the toys? Will the toys be accessible for the child once they start walking? Where will you keep the pram or stroller? Do you have a countertop for the steriliser, medicines, supplements and other items?

Space for the child, space for the child's belongings and space for you to grow with your child.

Despite the growing clamour around minimalism, first-time parents tend to not just go overboard but also end up getting way more than they need as gifts. Organising your stuff requires space, and if you don't have enough space, it will be a headache. Also, once the novelty of the child wears off, you will need space for your own breaks. It can be overwhelming to constantly be around the children, and breathing room is absolutely necessary. Therefore, you should consider these things before you're pregnant as far as possible.

If moving to a more spacious home is not an option, you need to work better with the space available to you. Bring out your creative hat and start thinking of alternative ways to use your space better. Work on maximising the utility of every corner of your home. Minimalism will aid the process, but you might want to get help redesigning your home if you aren't able to figure it out for yourself.

If you have a one-bedroom-hall-kitchen kind of set-up in a metro, think about how to not only maximise your space utilisation but also plan it in such a way that you don't lose your sanity within your own home. Plan such that while you get tons of storage, your home doesn't become cluttered or claustrophobic. It will need to become a smart combination of functionality and your preferred aesthetic. Some of the things you can do are:

- ✳ Get rid of stuff that hasn't been used for a year or more. If it hasn't been used for so long, it's rather unlikely that you'll be using it any time soon.

*   Try to redo your existing cabinets to make more functional partitions that will allow you to use every inch of available space.

*   Stuff that doesn't get used regularly but is required should be retired to the loft.

*   If you have beds, sofas, and cabinets with space underneath them, replace them with ones that have built-in storage.

*   If that's working out too expensive, get pull-out storage bins that can be used to store things like toys, diapers, extra bedding, etc.

*   The lower shelves of your cupboards should ideally be replaced with drawers to help you access things better, especially when the pregnancy is underway. Believe me, it's really difficult to bend down or squat too much to reach into the depths of the bottom-most shelves at 8-9 months.

*   Whenever you are looking to buy stuff for the baby or the mommy, try and get things that are multi-functional. For example, toys that have only one type of usage or that are unlikely to engage a child for long should be avoided. Get a diaper-changing bag that can double up as an overnight bag so that it's not a waste once the baby gets older.

*   Wherever possible, borrow things that are expensive or not frequently used, whether from friends, family, or a library.

*   See if you have empty space in any part of the house that can be converted into a half bedroom or nursery.

*   Also, please ensure you accommodate a desk or a small little office somewhere in your house if you're planning to work from home.

The bottom sections of all the cupboards in my house have drawers or pull-out storage. I just don't believe in digging into the back of a deep shelf and ruining the folding of a pile of clothes in the process. Also, I never did fancy sitting on the floor during my pregnancies. Sitting down at 9 months is hard, but getting up is really a challenge! I don't regret spending on the channels and wicker baskets that adorn my closets today.

These are super-pro tips from someone who's been through the cycle thrice. Paying attention to detail is key. Some of these smaller things will help make your life more organised and comfortable and reduce difficulty in adapting to your new lifestyle.

If you really want a bigger home and need to plan your finances for it, you had better start as early as you can. Factor in not only your current lifestyle and expenses but also the incremental expenses of pregnancy and the child. If this is going to be your first owned home, then it might be harder if you haven't saved up enough. These are big decisions to make and come at a huge cost, not just monetary but also psychological. Be prepared.

A friend of my husband's is a fantastic graphic designer. His business suffered badly during the recession as advertising expenditure of FMCG companies fell. They wanted to buy a bigger home using the money he and his wife had saved up through the first decade of their relationship, but their finances took a huge hit in the aftermath of the pandemic. While housing prices also fell, they didn't see their business recovering quickly enough to support them through the next 2 years when they would've ideally liked to have bought their new home and plan their second child. A home was something they couldn't give up on. So, they found an apartment that came cheaper than their current one in a different locality so that they could have more space as well as better infrastructure like gardens, swimming pools, etc.

We no longer live in homes with backyards and gardens for most part (I really envy you if you do!). This means we need to pay attention to our surroundings. If you live in a complex that has a decent playground and some open spaces, you're fortunate. If not, you need to look for these in the vicinity of your home. The open air is as important for the parents as it is for the child. I realised after having my eldest child that the open air makes a child far hungrier than the limited confines of my home. Seriously, nothing works like some cycling or running in the park to make a cranky child calm, a fussy eater hungry at mealtime, and a hypnophobic two-year-old fall asleep in a jiffy! After struggling for hours to put her to sleep, we would just take her for a small stroll in the garden and she'd invariably fall asleep on the way back. In the process, we would also feel de-stressed; not to mention relieved!

We'll discuss the financial planning for the baby in the coming chapters, but be rest assured, these are a few basic steps in the right direction. These questions may sound weird right now or too premature, but they are aimed at helping lay the foundation of your family. Did it ever cross your mind that having a baby would need so much of thinking? I'm sure not. That's because people everywhere still look at family planning as figuring out when to have intercourse to get pregnant. No denying you can't get pregnant without doing that, but is that all there is to 'planning a family?' Now you know, most certainly not.

Getting these things out of the way will also ensure that you are able to focus your energies on yourself and your family when the pregnancy is actually underway and you are under a lot of pressure. The decisions keep coming. The more you know and prepare for, the less you have to eventually worry about.

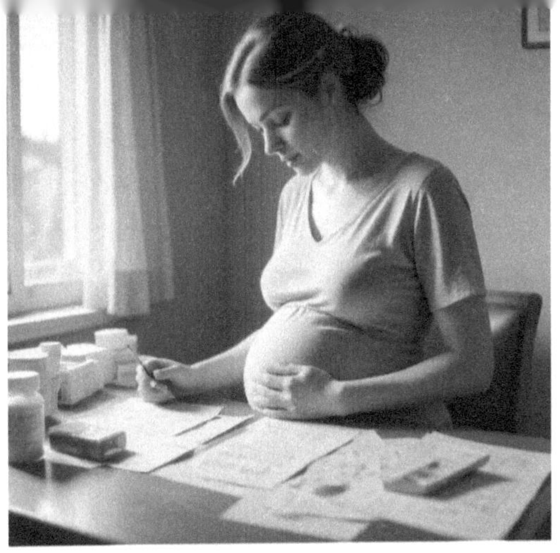

Chapter 5

BASIC BIOLOGY OF BECOMING PREGNANT

My story isn't a perfect ride. I had an unplanned pregnancy exactly a year after marriage. Although I wasn't mentally ready for the baby, there was no reason to not go through with the pregnancy. We had just returned from a holiday in Ladakh when we learnt about it, but the foetus stopped growing around 6 weeks and I had a missed abortion. It was an emotionally painful experience for me. I kept crying at the drop of a hat and there was this sense of loss that I couldn't define. Even my mom, someone who's always been so close to me and such a big pillar of support in the worst of times, couldn't actually fathom the depths of my pain. I can't blame her; she had never been through it and she may have been trying to keep me from focusing on it.

After the missed abortion, I found I became rather desperate to conceive again. It had happened naturally and suddenly the first time, so I thought I would be able to conceive quickly again. But all the stress of wanting it to happen meant that the 2 pink lines on the home pregnancy kit evaded me for many months. It started to unnerve me to even do the test.

I finally spoke to Dr. Salvi, who told me to just relax and let it happen when it should. Frankly, at that point, I wasn't sure whether she was just pacifying me or what, but I guess because she was such a senior doctor and she put me at ease in a snap, I tried to take her advice! Eventually, I found that the advice worked. A year after the miscarriage, I got busy with my younger brother's wedding. It was a huge event in my life that I had looked forward to forever and I plunged myself into the shopping and planning. All this took my mind off the stress of trying to get pregnant and unbeknownst to me, my mind relaxed enough to cooperate with my body! I actually conceived without trying too hard and was pregnant a month after his wedding!

Each person's journey is different. Someone may conceive easily and someone else may really struggle to get there. If you've been reasonably healthy and don't have any known health issues, you don't need to go to a doctor at the outset itself. You can try for as long as a year before you need to start worrying. If you tell your mother or grandmother that you are actually reading a book like this, they'll tell you that something is wrong with the kids nowadays. In their times, having a baby was a very natural extension of marriage and ideally happened within a year of getting hitched. And you only went to the doctor when you were close to the delivery date or if you were having some kind of problems in your pregnancy. That's clearly not how things work these days.

Pregnancy is about a complex system that is your body, which does include your mind. The human body is a massive set-up with such minute systems within systems that go haywire for the least probable reasons. Sex is only part of the process of conception. A mother's body needs to be prepared for receiving the seed of a new being and then, after the mating happens, it needs to be capable of nurturing that being.

Ideally, if everything is alright, people conceive within 12-6 months of trying. Studies conducted in the US say that about %90 of couples conceive within a year of trying while %95 of couples manage to conceive within 2 years of trying. So, it makes sense to keep an eye on your period cycle and keep trying for at least a year before you go to the doctor. If things haven't panned out by then, it doesn't mean that you will not be able to conceive. Rather, it means that you may have some small problems or may need some specific advice to help you conceive. To give you context, I want to point out that as per the same study, even out of the %5 of couples who don't conceive within 2 years of trying, %96 manage to get pregnant with the help of medical aid.

A visit to the doctor will help you understand why it isn't happening. It could be as simple as that you are not trying frequently enough or trying during the wrong part of the month. It's actually pretty common for couples to not know that you can't get pregnant by trying on just about any day. I, for instance, wasn't actually aware that it matters when you have sex to get pregnant! I only got to know when we started trying consciously that there's such a thing as ovulation. In high school biology, they teach you why periods happen, not how to avoid them!

So, learn about your period cycle. If you or your partner has regular periods, then it is easier to plan the intercourse in order to get pregnant. The key word here is "ovulation." Ovulation is the process of releasing an egg from the ovary. If your period is regular and your ovaries are working fine, ideally you should ovulate around 14 days from the first day of your last period. From there, the eggs are alive for around 36-24 hours and this is your window to get pregnant. You should start trying around a couple of days before your ovulation date as this is generally considered your most fertile period. The image below will help you understand the cycle better.

If your periods are irregular, it can be harder to predict when ovulation will occur. PCOS (Polycystic Ovarian Syndrome) is one of the major causes of irregular cycles in women. Statistics suggest that almost %20 of women in India suffer from PCOS. If you know you have PCOS, then start treating it with consistent lifestyle changes before considering medication. Medication may or may not be necessary to help you treat it, but rectifying your habits will be mandatory. You don't even need to keep running to doctors for the latter. There are plenty of apps and websites that can help you figure out how to improve your health, whether it's rectifying your diet or exercising.

If either you or your partner have fertility issues, you will need expert help. While some of these problems could result from your lifestyle, many may be entirely natural. This shouldn't mean that you are infertile or incapable of conceiving. As mentioned before, out of the %5 who don't conceive within 2 years, %96 do manage to get pregnant after receiving medical help.

While being at a healthy body weight is not necessarily a prerequisite for having a baby (I would know, as I bordered on the wrong side of the scale at the beginning of each one of my pregnancies), it can help, especially if you have other health conditions. The focus should not be solely on losing weight but on becoming healthy overall. Since people have different body types, what their bodies are capable of enduring also differs. Your focus should be on holistic health improvement rather than just the weighing scale. As part of your overall health check-up, the doctor will also ask you to get your blood pressure, blood sugar, and thyroid tested. The medical relevance of each is discussed in the section below.

Expert Speak
Hypertension

Hypertension, or high blood pressure, can affect a woman before pregnancy (chronic hypertension) or may arise during pregnancy (pregnancy-induced hypertension). If a mother has high blood pressure, it tends to worsen as the pregnancy progresses. Certain antihypertensive medications are not preferred during pregnancy as they may have adverse effects on the baby. Therefore, if a woman consults her physician before she becomes pregnant, the doctor will try to switch to safer antihypertensive tablets.

It may also lead to Pre-eclampsia. Pre-eclampsia is a condition where high blood pressure is accompanied by swelling of the feet and body along with the loss of protein in the urine. It generally occurs in the later part of pregnancy. All of this can affect the blood supply to the baby, causing growth restrictions. Thus, when a mother has high blood pressure, the doctor needs to control the same with safe medications and simultaneously monitor the health of both the mother and the baby.

Diabetes

Diabetes or increased blood sugar can affect a woman before pregnancy, or it may come up for the first-time during pregnancy. If it starts during pregnancy, it is called gestational diabetes. Diabetes can be dangerous for both the mother and the baby. The mother will have an increased predisposition to infection. Moreover, there may also be a higher chance of high blood pressure during the pregnancy. Both these factors together increase the chances of a caesarean section, especially when, due to diabetes, the size of the baby is larger when the maternal sugars are not well controlled.

Uncontrolled diabetes is associated with a higher chance of malformations in the baby. Blood sugars have to be well controlled before the pregnancy to prevent this increased risk of anomalies.

Babies of diabetic mothers tend to be overweight if the maternal sugars are not well controlled. Though they are big, they can have a host of problems, including immature lungs and respiratory distress at birth. They are not able to control their body temperature well and are also unable to control their sugar levels correctly. If the mother controls her sugars properly, the chances of the baby having a complication are reduced.

Knowledge is empowering in more ways than one. Being aware helps you not only do things better but also prevents you from falling prey to misinformation and blind faith. Especially with regard to something considered as sacred in our country as pregnancy, it is very easy to get carried away by old wives' tales and the mumbo-jumbo around fertility. Rest assured, the very fact that you are reading about something that was hitherto completely taken for granted by all is itself a step in the right direction for you and will help you to be more practical and successful in your endeavour to build a family of your own.

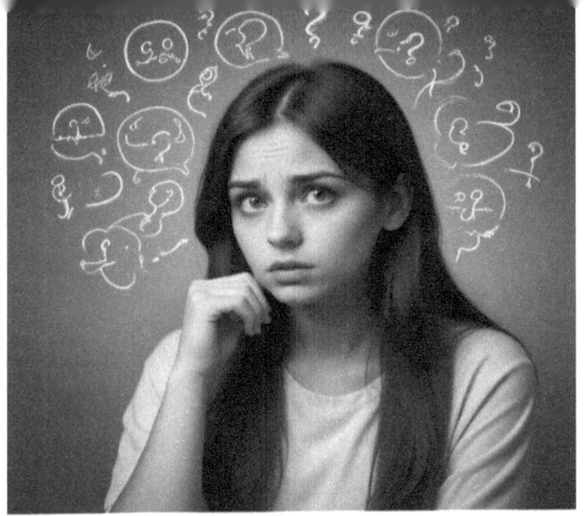

Chapter 6

CONDITIONING THE MIND

The day Tasha was born, her father refused to even hold her. The nurse brought her to him, expecting him to immediately take her in his arms. After all, he had been jumping in joy when he was told that it's a baby girl. But no, that wasn't the case. Tarun was scared shitless. He had never held a baby in his life. Not his friends,' not his neighbours,' no one's. And now, at that very moment, when he had become a father, the act of actually carrying the baby he had desperately been waiting to meet was so alien and scary for him that he just couldn't do it. He was scared he would drop her or carry her wrong and end up hurting her or something! It wasn't until Sharon actually came to and cajoled him into it that he finally carried his own child! That scene is forever etched in my mind though. The first meeting of 2 people who would forever be in love with each other!

When my husband's nephew was born, I realised that I hadn't seen a baby in the family in 20 years, let alone actually dealt with one. My husband though was an experienced hand who had watched his cousins raise their own children and had also played a role in the lives of his nieces and nephews. He was pretty good with children of all sizes, whereas although I was self-admittedly fond of children, I hadn't dealt with any newborns almost ever.

I got to hold our nephew, change his nappies, watch the *maalishwali maasi* (masseuse) massage him with almond oil (that my father-in-law would proudly get made first-hand from a cold presser), and even sing him lullabies. Some of it came naturally to me, but I don't think that's the case with everyone. I was lucky to get the whole low-down on baby-handling beforehand, at least to a limited extent. While caring for someone else's child is surely not the real deal, it does at least give you some sense of how to handle one.

Like Tarun and me, if you haven't had significant prior experience in being around children, it is important that you start preparing yourself mentally. It's not just about carrying the baby and changing diapers and soothing a crying child; it's about being comfortable in the knowledge that you are a parent and that you can be a good one. Even though you may not know how to do it all, just the acknowledgement of the role you are about to play is critical and to help you reach that state of self-acceptance will need some work. If you have an ecosystem that can help you prepare for your new role, great. If not, don't despair. There are a lot of options out there that you can explore.

If you don't already know extensively about them, prenatal and parenting classes are actually a thing.

Being a first-time parent is quite an overwhelming and intimidating feeling. You may walk in with the confidence of a pro but end up feeling like a complete failure within your first few minutes. It doesn't usually work by the book; it's more like a real-life GPS that keeps recalculating! Taking the aid of every external agency that can help you prepare better or improve your systemic responses to any minor crisis is not just advisable but, in my own experience, absolutely necessary.

There is a plethora of such classes available these days. Prenatal classes are very helpful, especially if you don't have any elderly or experienced person at home to guide you and show you the ropes of caring for the pregnant lady and preparing for the future. Some of the good things that you can pick up with respect to the pregnant woman at these classes include:

* Guidance on nutrition.
* Everyday do's and don'ts.
* Exercises to help strengthen the back and abdomen.
* Exercises helpful for long-term health.
* Guidance on mental health.
* Advice on how to plan your schedule.
* Advice on preparing for the baby.
* Shopping lists for the mother and child.
* Different types of childbirths.
* Enabling you to choose what works for you.

These things might seem a little excessive and random, but there's a good reason for learning them. Because we don't really get into this kind of role with significant experience and there are lives at stake, it is better to be careful and know especially what not to do. While you should always exercise your own discretion before following another person's advice, it is important to at least create a source of sound advice for yourself if you don't have one already. Even if you do have guidance at home, since things have changed so much in the domain of childcare and rearing in the past decade, it might be useful to still learn from updated experts. The simplest example of this is that our parents had no access to something modern parents can't live without – diapers. My own mother was really hesitant when

I told her how often my baby would wear diapers and it wasn't until my brother (who lives with my parents) had his first child that she understood how useful they are!

Other than teaching about caring for the pregnant lady, these classes can be very helpful if you haven't had any prior experience in baby care. They teach you about things like:

* How to hold the baby.
* How to change diapers.
* Checking temperature.
* How to bathe and clean the baby.
* Basic medical care and nutrition.
* How to nurse the baby.
* What to expect during the first few months.
* Best practices to ensure that you transition into the parenting role a little more easily; etc.

While it's wrong to say that these classes are enough, at least they give you a starting point and help you tackle complete ignorance and/ or lack of experience. One thing I can tell you after 3 kids is that no matter how much someone coaches you or tries to teach you about being a parent, what works for someone else may or may not work for you. You can try to adopt best practices learnt from those around you or things you read off the web, but the bulk of your knowledge will come while learning on the job. It does help, though, to improve your ability to cope with what can be controlled. That's why I do recommend reading up as much as you can and taking these classes because through a well-chosen class in your own locality, you can also create a great support network for yourself that will go through the problems that you go through at the same time.

My own experience is a case in point. Feeding my eldest a full meal until she turned 2 was the hardest thing I did on any given day.

Breakfast would be a task to be attempted at half-hour intervals from 8:30 am to 10:30 am and then finally giving up. The same would follow for lunch and then snack time and again dinner. I was on the verge of a breakdown. I was giving her semi-solid food which I thought would be easy for her to eat and included a lot of dense nutrition that the paediatrician said she needed. I tried every toy I could buy, every storybook she loved and for a couple of weeks, I also tried giving her my mobile phone to watch junk YouTube videos for toddlers. Nothing worked.

Then one fine day, a second-time mom from my pregnancy support group suggested that I try giving her the food we eat, in a similar plate and at the same time as us. I was really dubious as to how something this simple could work but she convinced me to try it and voila! It worked! For the first time in 3 months, she ate almost her entire meal and that too without throwing a tantrum. For every bite I ate, I would put a small bite in front of her and she would just mimic me and eat it as well. It was slow work because she took time to chew the food, but it was working! A lot of my friends have similar stories but all we will tell you is that it does get better and you should listen when people share their experience, rather than just random advice.

If you're not keen on all of this concentrated and focused advice, it's alright. Each unto his own. You might still want to make sure you get some form of good exercise and try prenatal yoga or Lamaze if it excites you. Again, if this stuff is not available in your vicinity or not your cup of tea, at least try learning some stuff off YouTube or ask your local yoga teacher for pregnancy-specific exercises. Meditation will also be most helpful and should be incorporated into your daily schedule.

When a baby is born, the nurses in the maternity ward usually do help you learn the first few basics like how to hold the child while breastfeeding, etc. But since that guidance is, firstly, available only for a couple of days, and secondly, very limited, you would do well to get help from other professionals. After doing these prenatal yoga and training classes, the process will still seem difficult but at least, you will have a vague idea of what you're supposed to do. The number of arguments couples can have over leaked diapers and badly swaddled babies is not funny. While these things may seem inane right now, believe me, when the time comes, diaper-changing and swaddling skills are something to be prized in parents-to-be. I know a distant cousin of mine asked a potential suitor what he thought of changing diapers when they were trying to get to know each other and was suitably impressed when he said he'd changed his sister's kid's diapers a few times!

Get your partner on board with the idea of attending some of these classes to not just learn the basics of child care but also to get into the parenting mood. It just helps to start training your conscious mind for the days to come and makes you feel a little better about yourself because you've prepared. It's like being in a flight simulator before you hit the runway full throttle! So yes, while it may feel like a stretch going for these things, really, there's nothing to lose. You might as well learn a thing or 2 while you can.

That's you and your partner. Then there's the ecosystem.

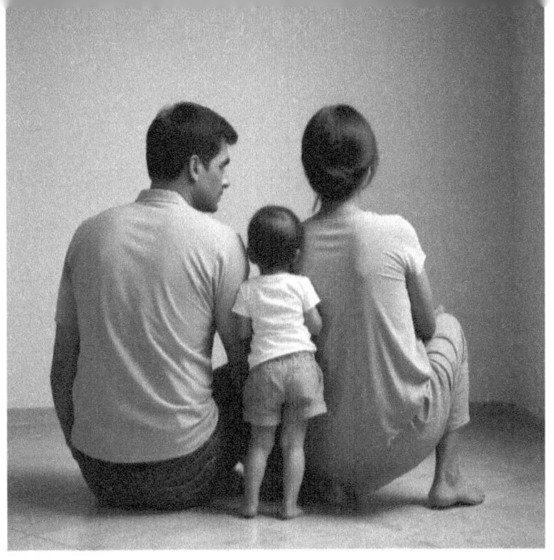

Chapter 7

THE FAMILY SUPPORT SYSTEM

Shalini is the youngest of 4 siblings. She was always the one everyone doted on and was not really used to making all her decisions on her own. She found the love of her life in college, and it was probably the only choice that was vetted by her parents long after it was made. After her father passed away, although all of her siblings were more than willing to have her mother live with them, Shalini insisted on her mother living with her and benefitted greatly from it. Had it not been for her mother's care, she might not have gotten through her rather complex pregnancy, further complicated by the long absences of her husband, a decorated Army Captain.

Not everyone's story is about having to give to their elderly or dependents. For a lot of people, the comfort factor in their lives is highly dependent on the support of their parents. If you live with your parents or in-laws (it's also possible that they're living with you), they will be an integral part of the child birthing and rearing process. They are experienced, tend to be patient and can provide a huge support system under the right conditions. If you share a good relationship with them, like in Shalini's case, it could be a most rewarding phase in all your lives because you will soon realise that some things are better done with the love and support of others than alone.

Most parents are extremely thrilled when they hear that a baby is on the way. It is a feeling they treasure and a phase of life they look forward to. Old age is difficult and having a little baby around can add a spark of joy to otherwise dull days. If your elders are not dependent on you in any way, they have more to give than to receive. You'd do well to bear in mind that they are in no way obligated to do anything for you, and it would be generous of them to spare time and effort to help you in your journey.

One has to take into consideration many things with respect to the elderly that you live with while planning your family. If your parents/in-laws are well and capable of taking care of themselves, they are likely to play a very helpful part in your pregnancy. By virtue of their experience of not only parenting but life in general, they would have invaluable advice to share. Even if you don't necessarily agree with the advice, be kind in your handling of it. Sometimes, all they want is to be heard out. Saying "Ok, let me think about it." is easier than getting into an argument.

The old tend to repeat the same thing many times, and it will get on your nerves or add to your anxiety. But just as you would be patient with your children, it is your duty to be patient with your ageing parents. Do this for them but also for yourself. It will not be entirely without selfish motive. Your parents will be a critical part of your lives and those of your children's if you can find the right balance of being dependent on them and allowing them to be dependent on you.

I know for a fact that my kids' life would have been far different and much less beautiful if not for their grandparents. Moreover, I can never imagine the kind of opportunities I have today if not for their presence. It is their presence that allows me to leave the kids home with the paid help under their supervision rather than a day care. Above all, the bond that children share with their grandparents is very special and rewarding for all.

I'm not saying it's always hunky-dory. Living with parents also means I have the added responsibility of not just caring for their health but also being emotionally available for them in the twilight of their lives. While they're still quite young and fit, they are increasingly dependent on my husband and me for things beyond their daily needs and must be handled patiently.

My in-laws weren't really a part of the discussions on pregnancy because it is such a big given in traditional families, but when I did eventually tell them about being pregnant, they were really thrilled. I mostly didn't agree with their thought process on pregnancy and pregnant women, but I had long learnt that hearing them out and then still making my own choices is far better than telling them that I disagree openly. I know this is not how the world is expected to work in the 21st century, but some things don't need to change. Relationships continue to be complex, and people's emotions and egos are as fragile as ever. The 'live and let live' attitude is better practised silently rather than belligerently. Therefore, a dash of conventional relationship management and silence combined with still making your own choices should make for a successful mantra!

Do your in-laws have a great say in your decision-making? Do they expect to be obeyed unchallenged or interfere with the decisions more than you expect? If so, you must be walking on eggshells all the time. As irritating and painful as that is, you must be in a position where you can't take on the in-laws head-on. You must both be allies of each other in the struggle of life before you have the strength to confront external forces. If your relationship is really terrible and you cannot find a functional median, then you may have to find a way to let the distance keep you civil with each other. In all other cases, cooperation through balanced understanding and some degree of compromise will make everyone's lives easier. If you live in different places, then it's not a matter of much discussion even.

If your equation with your in-laws is strained, it can cause undue stress in your relationship with your partner as well unless you both have the same reasons for the strain. It's critical that you both have common ground and know where each one of you needs to step back if there is a disagreement. This is especially relevant to ensure that when the ambient relationships are complex, it doesn't eat into your space and ruin the premise of your togetherness. Attain clarity on what you want and try to ensure that you both want more or less the same things. If you both want different things or want to do things drastically differently, under the added burden of the strained peripheral relationships, your own will surely suffer.

If you know how to function with your partner and vice versa in times of dispute, it would enable you to solve problems TOGETHER. You will learn about each other's strengths and where each one of you must take the lead. Maybe you could try to figure out a strategy between the 2 of you on how to tackle sticky topics with your family to reduce conflict. That way, less energy would be wasted, and you would be better equipped to actually do the deed.

Since I lived in a huge joint family kind of set-up, one of the hardest things for me was keeping personal things personal. Where I came from, other than my parents and brother, no one was ever consulted on a decision, and all information was passed on a need-to-know basis. Here, things were just the opposite. Initially, even if you sneezed, the whole family would know! Keeping something as big as a pregnancy secret until the third month was unimaginable! The first time I got pregnant, we made the mistake of going public with the news as soon as we found out. The excessive focus on the pregnancy was a killjoy. The second time around, we got wiser and told people after the third month. Since we had been through one experience together, we both agreed that even if the elders in the family were upset that we hadn't told them about the pregnancy early enough, eventually they would come around and wouldn't mind as much because of the prior experience we had had. The key here lies in 3 things:

- ✳ **Past experience** - we both had been through an experience in which we had learnt something together.

- ✳ **Learning from the experience** - we agreed that we should learn from our experience and not repeat our mistake.

- ✳ **Consensus** - we were willing to bear the consequences of our choice TOGETHER without blaming each other.

These are lessons that will hold you in good stead in your relationship in the long run, not just while planning the baby. Work on building the foundation of your family by communicating and trying to find middle ground. Remember to put each other first. Never make the mistake of putting others before each other. Eventually, you will only have each other to go through the journey of life. Even the children will grow up and have their own lives. If you don't build an understanding and the thought process that you must both be happy in whatever you do together, you will be on shaky ground always.

Another possible scenario is that the elders in your family are not particularly supportive of your having a baby or are dependent on you for health reasons. If they are not supportive at all and you need them more than they need you, you will have to find a way to convince them to throw their weight behind you and anchor you in your choice. If that's not working out, you will need to figure out how to become independent of them. If it's simply not possible, you may be looking at a stalemate that could turn painful.

If the elderly are dependent on you due to medical reasons, you need to plan not just for the baby but also to extend your support system to help you take care of all the dependents. You have to evaluate how your system would work in the future and come up with a strategy to ensure your resources are not stretched. A pregnant lady in the house means not just one hand less to perform its duties, it also means more work. Pregnant women need a fair amount of care and attention, especially if the pregnancy is happening later in life or if it's a complex case. Both of you will need to figure out who the primary caregiver of the family will be when the pregnancy is underway. The person has to be capable not only physically but also able to mentally handle the pressures the job will exert.

Another piece of the puzzle is the money. Take a look at how the finances will work during the period of the pregnancy and thereafter. If the mother-to-be was the primary caregiver of the elderly/dependents in the family, she may either have to stop working for a while to be able to deliver on her responsibilities or hire an additional hand to take care of the dependent(s). Either way, your finances will be affected. You will have to save up enough to meet these exceptions in your cashflow before you plan the pregnancy. If that's no longer an option as the pregnancy is underway, you will have to find a way to rework your finances.

A dear friend of ours was in a situation where his mother was diagnosed with cancer during his wife's second trimester. Since he's an architect, he had to cut back on work to be able to take his mom for the chemotherapy sessions and help with her day-to-day care. This hit their finances in the short term. They sold off their luxury sedan, which had a -6figure EMI, to get a smaller car and reduce their EMI burden. It wasn't a big sacrifice, but it helped reduce stress in the short term.

For families with elderly who have some kind of disability or degenerative condition, the talk of a baby can be daunting. I have a friend whose mother-in-law was bedridden due to a slip disc surgery gone wrong. She had to give up her full-time job as an air hostess with an international airline as there was no one else to help care for her MIL. She had planned on switching careers as it is but had to do it earlier than planned as a result of this. When she got pregnant, the struggle was pretty bad because they had not planned for anything. They had to get paid help in her second trimester as she could no longer lift her mother-in-law to bathe her or feed her, and the physical care of a bedridden patient is definitely not something a pregnant woman can cope with. Added to that, she had a low-lying placenta because of which her doctor advised her extensive bed rest in her last trimester.

Expert Speak

Seema got up in the middle of the night sensing that her gown was wet. She was seven months pregnant. She got really alarmed when she saw that blood had trickled out of her vagina and soaked her gown and bed sheet. Her family immediately rushed her to the hospital. An emergency ultrasound revealed that her placenta (the organ that connects baby to mother) was located right over the mouth of the uterus. Normally the placenta is attached to the mother's uterus at the upper part of the uterine cavity. Occasionally it attaches and implants on the lower segment. If it is located just above or close to the internal os (internal opening/mouth) of the uterus, it is termed placenta previa. In such cases, the mother can present with painless bleeding, which is what Seema also had.

The diagnosis of placenta previa is confirmed by ultrasound. If there is bleeding before the baby is mature, the doctor tries to conserve the pregnancy. However, if the bleeding worsens, the mother will need to be delivered irrespective of the baby's maturity. If there is no or minimal bleeding, the pregnancy is conserved up to term. At term, the baby needs to be delivered by a Caesarean section, since the placenta which is covering the os (internal opening/mouth) of the uterus, prevents the baby from delivering normally.

This story is proof that you need to think ahead if you have such a situation in your family. That doesn't mean you must be deprived of the joy of having a child, but you need to plan better to ensure that the family doesn't undergo undue strain because of it. Finding good help is one of the keys. You will need to get extra hands-on-board and make sure you are well-equipped for the extra work. Caring for a special needs family member is difficult, and so is going through a pregnancy. The last thing you want is to be struggling to cope with both. Better to build your backup mechanisms in advance.

Please remember that everything that goes wrong is just one extra reason for both of you to get into a fight. As if relationships aren't complex enough already. So, plan. I can't stress enough the role that planning will play in every stage of your life. The number of times I get asked how I can look so peppy on most days despite 3 kids and a career is not funny. The biggest reason I'm surviving is because we chose to enlist help and trained them enough to handle tasks that can be delegated. When people ask me how I cope with it all, I only tell them one thing – I run my home like people run a business. I have a weird acronym, READ to achieve this:

- ✳ **Roles** – define what roles need to be fulfilled and what skills are needed to accomplish them.

- ✳ **Enlist** – find the right people to fulfil these roles and delegate tasks to them.

- ✳ **Automate** – whether it's bill payments, auto-ordering of regular medicines or as basic as using calendar reminders on your phone, automate everything you can.

- ✳ **Deliver** – focus your energies and deliver on the things that only you must do or that only you can do.

Your tasks could be cooking, cleaning, paying bills, ironing clothes, walking the dog, buying groceries and so on. When I talk about getting help, I mean finding people to do what out of these things others can do. Hire a cook to make a meal at least once a day, or find a good home-made tiffin service. Hire a part-timer to come in and do the dishes, sweeping and swabbing. Automate your monthly bill payments. Start using online delivery services for your groceries instead of lugging them around. The more you delegate and automate, the more independently functional your home system will become. It will free up your time to care for that little human you're so keen to have in your life and still be able to spend time with those close to you!

Another thing that happens as a baby arrives is that your memory tends to suffer. My husband has said innumerable times that I'm just not the same person I was when we got married. From being someone who never forgot to do anything, to becoming someone who can't remember for the life of me why I came into the room, I've undergone a huge transformation. It's obviously not on purpose. While I'm told that the hormones have something to do with it, it's equally true that sleep deprivation and the never-ending list of things that are non-negotiable are highly responsible. Everyone except the baby is priority number 100! So, start using a planner and reminders on your phone. Some of the things that I found useful over time are:

* Apps to track credit card and bill payments.

* Auto-debit facilities for my monthly utilities.

* Apps that help track and order my groceries.

* Wearable devices to help care for my health better, including step count, reminders to drink water, reminders for medicines, etc.

* Recurring reminders on my phone for monthly appointments and meetings.

The same is applicable if you have an elderly person to care for. Get help if you must. Also, get your ward a wearable device that'll help remind them of their medicines and meals. Make sure you build a support system for them that allows them to spend their time happily rather than being completely dependent on you. We don't realise how much they need us. Every time we add a new responsibility to our life, the time we spend with our parents reduces. Also, our emotional bandwidth for dealing with them takes a hit with stress coming from other quarters. The least we can do is lessen the blow and help keep their lives full and happy even with our reduced availability. I'm not exaggerating. You don't want to feel guilty about it later, right? So why not put requisite systems in place now.

While your availability will be lesser, don't saddle yourself with guilt. You have a right to your life. Also, the little addition to your family will bring joy to your folks as much as she will to you. It's all for a good cause. You can make things move smoothly and ensure a seamless transition by being more perceptive and staying one step ahead of the curve.

I must reiterate at this time: it's true, it does take a village. If you think it's only about you and the baby, no it's not. You cannot be the sole caregiver; you will never be the only teacher, and you don't want to end up being the only source of love. The more people in your child's life, the fuller it is. It could be family; it could be friends. *Don't isolate yourself because loneliness doesn't make for a happy anything.* Take care of those around you and let them care for you while they can.

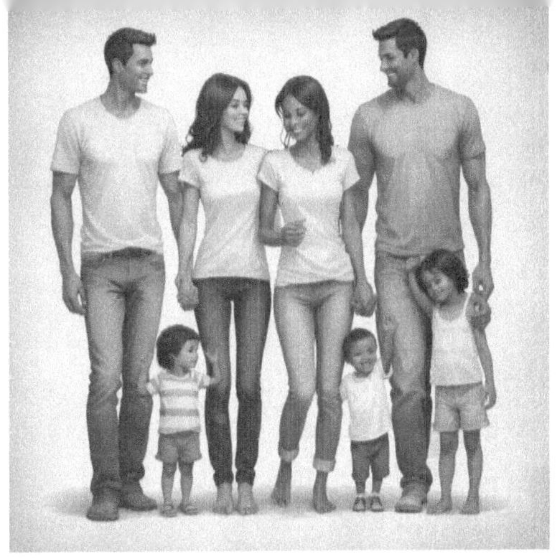

Chapter 8

THE BACKUP MECHANISM

Manisha was in her last trimester of pregnancy. Her mother wanted to make a trip to meet Manisha's brother living in London before her delivery as she knew she would not be able to make a trip for at least a few months after her daughter's delivery. So, her mother flew out, leaving Manisha at the mercy of their part-time helpers and friends. A few days into her stay in the UK, the pandemic hit, and all flights were grounded. Manisha's mom couldn't make it back until way after the baby was born. It was one trip she really regretted making.

But Manisha didn't suffer as much as her mother thought she would. She was practical and figured things out as best as she could. As soon as they got to know that all international flights were grounded and it didn't look likely that things would get better in a hurry, Manisha spoke to the agency from which she had intended to hire her jaapa maid and got them to send someone in advance. She was willing to spend the extra money to ensure that she didn't have to struggle. The jaapa not only ensured that she was taken care of well through the last phase of her pregnancy, but she also filled the void of experience left by Manisha's mother's absence.

Also, luckily for Manisha, since she lived in a large apartment complex, she had a lot of friends in the vicinity. So even in the days of panic stocking of groceries due to the pandemic, she didn't have to run around herself. Her friends would take turns to get her stuff and get through that dreaded period. All of this while her husband was stuck in Dubai where he had gone to complete a major project for his employers.

Pregnancy and parenting mean a lot of decisions. And every decision is literally life-changing. Did you even imagine when you set out on this journey that becoming a parent is not just about biological success? Or that you would have to think through a trillion things before you were considered worthy of being a good parent? If you're anything like me and most of my friends, probably not. I can write this book only in hindsight. I didn't possess even an ounce of this wisdom before I started. I may have gotten terribly lucky in many ways, but I don't deserve the credit for having known any of this before my eldest was born. The only good thing about the post-partum analysis is that I am now in a position to pass down all this accumulated wisdom!

Not all of us live with family or have relatives in the same city. Some of us don't even have relatives at all! Does that mean that you will never have a support system? Of course not! There are different elements of a support system for anyone in life, over and beyond your blood relatives. How you build that system or enhance the one you were blessed with is actually a question of 3 things. One, the realisation that you need help. Two, the willingness to ask for help. And finally, the effort of creating healthy, mutually beneficial relationships.

For many of us, especially those without extended families or those living away from their loved ones, our true support system comes from our friends. If you are one of those people, then you have hope. Your friends can play a huge role in every step of the pregnancy and baby-planning process and thereafter. This helps especially because friends tend to be less judgemental than family and are most often our peers. They're more likely to get us and have the same frame of reference, which is invariably missing in older family members. Even if your friends are in a different age group, that you are friends is a result of you both sharing the same wavelength.

If you are seriously considering a baby and have started planning the process, have you discussed it with your closest friend(s) yet? Unlike your mother who might nag you about it every day, your bestie is unlikely to harass you for a progress report on your pregnancy plans. He or she will also be more likely to understand the key factors determining your state and stage of life. Even if your bestie is someone who's more hyper than you are and is a bit of a nag, the saving grace is that you can still be yourself with them and probably get heard out. They know you well, get what you're going through and have the courage to call you out for any wrong choices you may be making! The best thing is that they would also understand your anxiety and the pressures you are dealing with. Don't hold back; take the leap of faith and offload.

If you haven't opened up to your close circle, is it because you're concerned about them having a different perspective on children than you? Even if that is the case, it's alright to open up. Sometimes, our friends see more clearly that which we don't. If you are on the fence regarding getting pregnant, or if either you or your partner is having doubts about how you both would fare as parents, it might be a good idea to involve your friends in a closed group discussion. Some of the key things you could discuss with them include:

* Do your friends see you as the parent-type? Do they think you have the parenting gene?

* Do they think you're financially ready for a baby?

* What's their take on the current status of your career?

* Do they think your career can handle the break for parenthood?

* Is it the right time for you emotionally?

* What is the advice they would give you on timing and preparation?

* Would they be able to support you in any way? E.g. going to the doctor, assisting you in your decision-making, enabling you to find help, providing support when one partner is travelling, etc.

If your friends already have children, they're a valuable source of not just information but also perspective. They will be able to provide insight into what worked for them and what didn't. Some of the things you can ask of your friends with children are:

* When did they know they were ready?

* How long did they try before they conceived?

* References of doctors

* What kind of money they had put aside before they seriously considered having children?

* What were the big changes in their lives after the kids came along?

* What should you be prepared for that they realised later?

* How they dealt with sticky issues, etc.?

We all value our privacy and want to keep our secrets to ourselves. Especially if we're having trouble with conception or if it's a touchy topic in our family, we are likely to become a bit reclusive and get into an emotional rut. Are you feeling the stress of going through all of this and find yourself unable to voice it out? Has restricting your emotional outlet to your partner increased the burden on them also? Then the easiest thing to do is to open up to your close friends. Even if your friends are yet to start a family or don't want to, they might not be able to give you advice but surely can hear you out. They can be your safe space and a source of comfort.

Talking to our close friend(s) helps dispel our feelings of loneliness and gloom. Our friends are the support system that demands far less of us than our family because that's what friends are – family without the strings. They have the ability to understand us better and share our mindset. They see through our silence and give us an ear when we need it the most. Don't shy away from speaking to them; it will really help. Also, remember, since they are unlikely to have a vested interest in your having a baby, they are more likely to give you an unbiased perspective and will not be as emotionally involved in your decisions as your partner.

Are you hesitant to involve your close friends in the process? Maybe you fear that they may be too busy, or you may be disturbing them unnecessarily. Try putting yourself in their shoes, and perhaps the act will become easier on your conscience. You will realise that if roles were reversed and your friend was going through a tough time, you would've expected them to approach you irrespective of your schedule!

Other than just the emotional and moral aspects, your friends can be a great source of practical support as well. Whenever your partner is unavailable to go to the doctor with you, enlist your friends' help. Not only will they be happy to go with you, but the fact that they have been with you through the process will help bring you all closer. Eventually, it'll also allow for your friend to have a special rapport with your children because they were part of the child's birth story.

It's good to have someone take care of you when you are at your most vulnerable. If your partner needs to make those visits in your absence, make sure you encourage your partner to not only take a friend along but also try to schedule the appointments with the gynaecologist when the friend is available. That way, even if the father is physically unavailable, he's involved in the process. Doing this will make your friends happier about helping you out and will ease your hesitation as well. After all, what are friends for!

Share your concerns with your buddies. It will help you reduce undue anxiety and paranoia. Being careful is good, but paranoia in times of conception or while pregnant does more harm than good. A good friend will be able to calm you down and help improve not just your state of mind but will be able to lend a helping hand when it matters. It could be finding more house help, assistance in paying bills, planning doctor's visits, going for check-ups, or just giving you company when you need it. Nothing a good friend can't do.

My husband has been to the doctor with me for every single appointment through my 3 pregnancies, barring one. Although he was so involved in the process, at times when we had a fight or were at loggerheads, I would just talk to a friend of mine who has always been good at cooling my temper off. He doesn't have kids and is unlikely to even get married, but is one of the most sorted people I've ever met. He would actually look at things very matter-of-factly and call me out if he thought I had behaved unreasonably. Although it's not like he was sharing personal experience, such a neutral perspective always did wonders for my state of mind. He helped me see my husband's side of the story often.

If you don't have this precious thing called a close friend, try and enlist the help of your friendly neighbours. If you have a good elderly neighbour who you know would be happy to help out, confide in them and tell them you need help. Like Dumbledore says, help will always be given to those who ask for it. If you don't ask, nobody knows you need any help, right?

In the long run, you and you alone are going to be responsible for building your support system. This will include your family, your friends, your neighbours, and your paid help. Don't inflate your sense of self by thinking you can be a one-person army. All it takes is one bad day for the sky to fall on your head and for not just your confidence but also your positivity to crash. You can't prevent the bad days but you can prevent the crash. Reduce your fragility and spread the eggs into various baskets. The more backup mechanisms you have, the easier it gets to deal with unexpected problems. The more the number of people you have on your speed dial, the better the chances that someone will turn up when it matters. In a real-life situation, it is impossible that the person you rely on the most will be available every single time you have a problem. But if you rely on a number of people, surely if one can't make it on time, another will!

Find options for everything. What kind of options, you ask? These examples will give you some insight:

* Transport - You'll need alternatives in case your regular means are unavailable. If you are used to self-driving or if your driver doesn't turn up, be ready to take a cab or have a friend who's willing to drive you over to the doctor's.

* Food - Find a good home-made tiffin service to help provide meals when you can't make yourself a meal or your cook hasn't turned up.

* Domestic Help - Make sure you are on good enough terms with a couple of part-time helpers in the building or area who can pitch in if your regular help doesn't turn up. You could also ask your regulars to ensure they designate temporary replacements who can fill in for them on holidays. There are also websites these days that send help who work by the hour and come at pretty short notice.

- ✳ Pantry - Start stocking your basics a bit on the higher side and maintain that buffer. Especially when it comes to things that you may end up craving in the middle of the night, nothing is too much. Believe me, a little extra stock to manage is better than a helpless or irate partner when you're having a bout of uncontrollable cravings!

- ✳ Medical help - If your obstetrician/gynaecologist is some distance off or doesn't give his/her own mobile number, make sure to have their assistant's contact number and also the number of a general physician who can help you out in an emergency.

- ✳ Emergencies - Make sure you have contacts of all repair services – from the cable to the washing machine, from the plumber to the electrician.

In this day and age of apps and home entrepreneurs, you have choices for everything at your fingertips. Make use of those. A lot of this sounds like common sense, but it's stuff we realise we should've done earlier only when the shit hits the ceiling. These things, though not strictly related to having a baby, are life-savers in the most unprecedented of situations. I must have been 8 months pregnant with my eldest, and my husband was out of the city for a day. I was alone at home, and the hinges on the main door came loose. I had a spare pair of hinges left from when we'd moved into the house, but our carpenter was travelling. I called our regular electrician, and he fixed the door. He just did it because we'd known him for so many years.

Building a support system is a process. It doesn't happen overnight. Also, it doesn't happen by just asking for favours. I mean, how would you feel about getting requests for help from someone who's never had a nice word to say to you for years? Start by being nice and offering to help when others need it. You rub my back, I rub your back. It's as simple as that. If you've done enough for people, they're far more likely to return the favour than if you turned a blind eye or turned down a request in someone else's hour of need. Also, remember, karma is always watching. You never know when you might need whom. These are life lessons, some learnt the hard way.

The one and only time I went for a doctor's appointment alone, it was July and it was pouring cats and dogs in Mumbai. No cabs were available, and the reason I had gone alone was that my husband had gone for a meeting (he'd taken the car) and had forgotten about the appointment. I was so mad at him that I didn't remind him about it and went off alone. As luck would have it, I got stuck there because of the rain. I took out my umbrella and was trying to hail a rickshaw. After about 20 minutes of waiting, a car stopped near me. It was my neighbour's sister who lived close by. She knew I was on good terms with her brother's family and gladly dropped me home. It couldn't have come at a better time.

So, yes. While taking pills and getting tests done and all is important, in the rush to get your life sorted, don't forget the people around you. They really, really do matter at the end of the day. Even if you don't finally need to call in a favour, knowing that if you ever need one, those people are there, is enough.

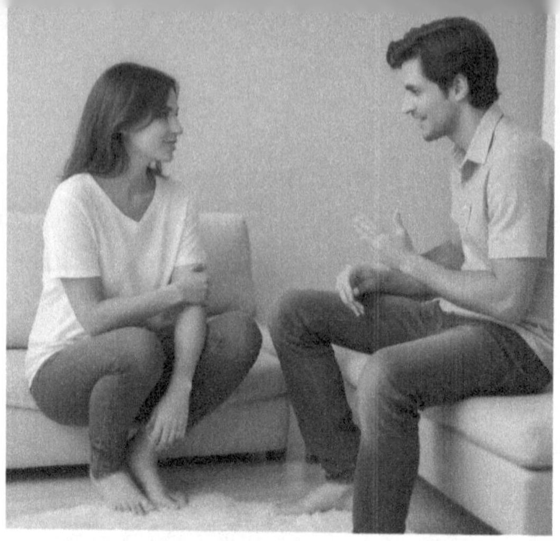

Chapter 9

THE CONCEPTION PROCESS

There's a quote from *The Fault In Our Stars* that goes like, "Grief does not change you. It reveals you." It was only after my miscarriage that I realised how important being a mother was to me. I knew I wanted to have a baby at some point, but the grief of losing that child made the want so tangible, it hurt.

I decided 6 months after to go see the doctor. She said there was nothing wrong with me and that since I had conceived naturally once, I would surely conceive again. Maybe I was just trying at the wrong time of the month! Whaaat??? Time of the month?!!! Whatever did that mean? And so, just like that, I realised that I actually knew very little about the conception process itself. I mean everyone on this earth knows how babies are born, right? Wrong. A lot of people live in some form of ignorance regarding how a baby is actually conceived; that there is something beyond the physical intimacy required between a man and a woman. And I happened to be one of them.

So, apparently, this is how it works. Once a month, a mature egg is released by one ovary in a woman's body. The process of releasing the egg is called ovulation. If intercourse happens around the time of ovulation and a sperm mates with the egg, it is said that the egg is fertilised. The egg and sperm combine to form a foetus, which then latches itself to the wall of the woman's uterus to start growing, and the woman is then said to have conceived.

Once you figure out when you want the baby, it's good to also learn about the finer details of what it takes to get pregnant. If you haven't heard horror stories of how people have had trouble getting pregnant, please acquaint yourself with some of them. If getting pregnant was that easy, like mentioned earlier in the book, there wouldn't be so many fertility clinics in the world. If you are reading this after having quickly conceived, you can just skip to the next chapter.

When a couple starts trying, there's a lot of pressure every month. It's like a cyclical repetition of the climax of some horror movie, with the chief protagonists hoping for a different end each time! First, you try and try and try, hoping that one day, the sperm will score. Then you start counting backwards to the period date. If the period arrives like an unwanted guest, it's a huge anti-climax, a terrible end to that run of the movie. If the period doesn't arrive, the tension peaks when you put 2 drops of urine on that little stick, which is reminiscent of the build-up to the end. A single pink line is an arrow through the heart; 2 pink lines are the elusive happy ending!

What pink lines am I talking about? The ones that appear on home pregnancy test kits. These kits cost around Rs. 50 per pack and help you to check whether you are pregnant, at home in the privacy of your bathroom. They come with a small plastic strip which has a tiny cavity on them. You put 2 drops of the first urine of the morning of the wannabe-mommy. The test works by checking for hCG, the pregnancy hormone in your urine. This hormone rapidly increases in your bloodstream as soon as you conceive and is at its peak around 10-8 weeks into the pregnancy. If there is hCG (human chorionic gonadotropin hormone) in your urine, there will be 2 pink lines on the test strip. If you see only one, it usually means that you are not pregnant. It is possible though that you may get a false negative on the test sometimes.

If you tested too early, then your 2 pink lines will not appear. You might want to wait a couple of weeks more so that there's enough hCG in your body. It's possible that even though you are pregnant, the body is not producing enough hCG to show on the test. So don't panic if there was just 1 pink line. It could be due to other reasons. If no lines show on the test kit after putting the urine drops, however, it means that your test didn't work right. You will have to do another one.

It's a terrible phase to go through. I can't tell you how much stress it meant to do the test. I remember dreading having to do it just for the fear of disappointment. If you're feeling the same way, please know that you are not alone. There are thousands, maybe lakhs, of people out there who are going through the same thing. The anxiety, the fear, the disappointment – it's only too common. It's difficult and unfair but there's not much you can do about it.

I can tell that eventually though, you will be fine. It will happen. One way or the other, you will not be deprived of the joy you so seek. When people tell you this, your acrimonious anger towards them is also justified. Sometimes even the people we are closest to don't appreciate the struggle this process is. Even people who have been through these struggles can be somewhat smug about it and make tactless jokes that are likely to rub you the wrong way. Don't expect empathy, don't expect them to understand. This is life and it is unfair. Keep it together and hang in there.

What you can do to aid you in your process is to use another home kit that, to some extent, helps plan your cycles. That's the ovulation kit. These kits help you figure out where you are in your cycle, especially if you have errant periods. This ensures you know when the best time is to have sex in order to get pregnant. Doctors don't generally recommend ovulation kits as they prefer that patients take the natural approach to conception. But just so you know, they do exist.

While nothing can guarantee you getting pregnant, I can tell you some of these things do help. Discuss between the 2 of you what you think the problem may be if there is one at all. Maybe taking the help of some over-the-counter aids like the ovulation kit can help you get results. It's entirely possible that even then, you may not get pregnant quickly. But the money involved isn't too large, and you can always give it a shot. If not, you start seeing a doctor.

For people who don't conceive even after a year of trying naturally, the doctor will ask you to go in for some tests. If the reports of these tests are fine but your cycles are irregular, the doctor may even suggest going in for a follicular study to help monitor the growth of the eggs in the woman's ovaries. If the growth of the eggs is fine, the doctor will help you plan your intercourse and tell you when your most fertile period for trying is. If the follicular study shows that the eggs are not growing to a good enough size to aid conception, they might give you hormonal pills to help the eggs grow better. Chances are that you might end up getting pregnant within a few follicular study cycles.

In some cases, the problem is not with the eggs. Men also suffer from fertility-related issues. One common one is sperm motility. Sperm motility is the ability of the sperm to move through the female reproductive tract in order to reach the egg. It is one of the parameters of the quality of the sperm because unless the sperm can swim through the body fluids to reach the eggs, there will be no fertilisation and hence pregnancy. If all is well with the lady, the doctor may ask the male partner to get their sperm tested. It can be remedied with some medication.

I do hope that you are now a little more acquainted with the pregnancy planning tools and processes than before. We tend to deal with a lot of anxiety because we fear the unknown. Arming yourself better with the basic knowledge of the process can help reduce your stress levels and potentially aid your conception process. Beyond that, this knowledge should also allow you to be open to seeking help should the need arise. All in all, at least now you know more than you did before.

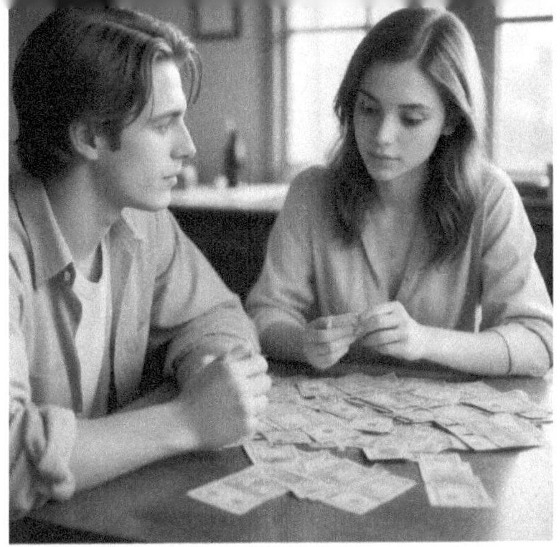

Chapter 10

PREPARING YOUR FINANCES FOR THE PREGNANCY

Kavita had been working with us as an accountant for nearly 6 years before she conceived her first and only child. Her husband works with a travel insurance company, and the 2 had worked really hard to build a life in a city as expensive as Mumbai. The large part of Kavita's salary went into the EMIs of their one-bedroom-hall-kitchen apartment in an upcoming locality on the outskirts of Mumbai. Her husband's salary took care of the other expenses and a small monthly savings scheme they had started putting money into early in their marriage. For a regular middle class Indian couple, they were really disciplined in how they handled their finances, and you would never find them splurging on anything unnecessary. Even then, when Kavita delivered their son and the hospital bills came, it nearly wiped out all the hard-earned money they had put into the liquid savings scheme.

The real pace of pregnancy is nothing like what you see in those dreamy ads or fantastical movies that talk about the beauty of being pregnant. It's a beautiful process that's not under your control, and its pace can be absolutely frantic and dreadfully dull at the same time. It is really a lesson in patience in a number of ways and is best enjoyed with a pinch of salt. And only with some amount of money in the bank.

While we've already spoken about some of the ways in which you would need to prepare yourself for the pregnancy, what we'll discuss here is how to work towards ensuring you earmark the right amount of money for the whole process. This kind of planning is critical in ensuring you don't get any shocks later on and are able to meet your own expectations more than anyone else's when the time comes. Like in the case of Kavita and her husband, even sound financial planning won't help if you don't estimate your delivery costs and the expenses thereafter correctly.

I always suggest that when you're thinking about the future, plan on the higher side. You don't know how lucky or unlucky you are going to be in this process. Everything may go smoothly, and you may not need to spend more than a few thousand on a few doctor's visits and the mandatory nutritional supplements. After all, a natural conception and an uncomplicated pregnancy are less expensive. Or you may be faced with some kind of delays and obstacles and may need medical intervention. This could cost anywhere between a few tens of thousands to a couple of lakhs. So, beware before you embark on this journey. Don't take the money involved lightly. Even if you don't need that much money through the pregnancy and for the delivery eventually, saving more than you needed will leave you better off in your personal finances.

My husband and I have spent a lot of money during our first couple of years of marriage on holidays because we're both travel buffs. However, we were prudent enough to put various forms of savings in place. This was primarily because although neither of our families traditionally went to well-known maternity hospitals, he was always particular about the kind of medical care he wanted for me and our baby. When we did our research, we found that a regular delivery at the hospital of our choice would cost us a little over Rs.1,00,000. This was back in 2013 and for a normal delivery.

We had savings in 2 liquid forms – fixed deposits and shares. We also started a recurring deposit after we found out I was pregnant to ensure that the money outflow wouldn't be sudden and wouldn't hit us in our business cash flows. If you run your own set-up, it is even more important for you to plan in advance because business can be unpredictable and such large expenses can impose a massive strain on your reserves.

What I would suggest to you is to split your cost over the period you intend to start trying after. Let's say you hope to be pregnant a year from now. You should ideally divide the cumulative cost of your pregnancy and delivery over the period of that one year. That's how long you have to set aside the money. If you've already been saving, then of course you won't have too much trouble continuing the trend. If not, start immediately. You can always opt for cheaper services but even the most cost-effective maternity homes these days do cost a fair amount.

The starting point for saving is knowing how much you are actually spending. Prepare a budget with your standard monthly expenses against your bare minimum monthly income. Ideally what is left should cover your regular savings and the amount you need to put away monthly for your delivery cost. If not, you would need to cut back on extravagances and unnecessary items. Needless to say, if both of you are earning, then you both should be sharing the burden. The best way to ensure this amount gets put aside is to start a recurring deposit account. You won't have to worry about remembering to do it, and the interest income will keep adding up as well.

It would help to discuss the overall approximate average figures for the cost of prenatal care at this point.

A pregnant woman requires certain medication and vaccinations which are mandatory. She may also have to undergo certain basic tests prescribed by the doctor. The monthly cost of these averages around Rs.2,000. So assuming she found out about the pregnancy in the second month, till the end of the eighth month, this is a total of 7xRs.2,000 per month, i.e., Rs.14,000.

In the initial phase of the pregnancy, you need to visit the doctor once a month. After the second trimester, i.e., from the seventh month onwards, you start going to the doctor twice a month. In the last month, you end up going every week. So on average, you would be visiting your doctor around 14-12 times in your pregnancy. At an average of Rs.500 per visit, this totals to Rs.7,000. If your obstetrician charges more, then you need to factor accordingly.

Next comes the cost of various sonographies that you must get done as per your doctor's advice. You could end up having to get as many as 8 done through the course of your pregnancy, and there could be a few recurring ones in the last month to ensure the baby is fine. Some of these tend to be expensive and cost an average of Rs.2,000 per scan. So that's a total of Rs.16,000 at the very least.

We've discussed in the previous chapters how the quality of our nutritional intake should improve, whether it is the father or the mother. This means adding more fruits, vegetables, and even sources of protein to your diet consciously. The average incremental cost of these in a tier1- city could be as high as Rs.3,500 per month. For 8 months, that works out to Rs.28,000.

We can total our expenses as follows:

Particulars	Average Cost for a Tier1- City (Rs.)
Medical expenses of the mother-to-be	14,000
Doctor's visits	7,000
Sonographies	16,000
Incremental food expenses	28,000
Total	65,000

I know it's strange that something as beautiful as pregnancy should be spoken about in money terms. But these are the practical facets of life. We can choose to ignore them, but it would be at our own peril. I have taken the bare minimum costs into consideration here. The cost of your prenatal care could go up or down based on your personal preferences and lifestyle. For example, some people go all out on a maternity wardrobe. An average maternity outfit can cost anywhere between Rs.-900Rs.1,800. For a minimum of 10 outfits that a pregnant woman would require, this alone is an additional Rs.18,000. If you opt for prenatal classes or pregnancy yoga or Lamaze classes, it could cost you a bare minimum of Rs.1,500 per month from the fourth month to the ninth. That's another Rs.9,000 added to the above figure.

One thing that I was sorely disappointed to find out was that my husband's family had no tradition of a godh-bharai or a baby shower. It's something I had always dreamt of, and when finally my time had come, I found out that we didn't do it! I was really, really upset about it. But my husband threw me a surprise birthday party cum baby shower with close friends and family. It was a wonderful gesture and something I will cherish forever.

If your family does have such a ceremony, then you might want to factor in that cost. Or if you intend to have a modern baby shower party, then you can take that into consideration. If you plan one by yourself with your family and friends, it can be quite cost-effective, and you would also end up getting some lovely presents to pamper the mother and the baby. I did find out how much my baby shower cost us (I handle the finances of the company and the family!). Just the party venue and food cost him about Rs.19,000. My sister-in-law pitched in with the games and decorations while his best friend's wife brought us the cake. If you take all that into consideration, the sum would be much higher. I have been to baby showers that have been planned on a really grand scale, and honestly, if you have that kind of money, go all out. Otherwise, be wise in what you choose to spend on!

So while there is a base calculation that one can do, there's no upper limit to what you want to and what you can spend on during the pregnancy. If we add all these incremental things and say your pregnancy is slightly more expensive than what I've considered, you could end up shelling out as much as Rs.1,50,000 during this period.

Each one of you needs to set aside half of that. If one of you makes a lot more than the other, you can do a pro-rata distribution of the money to be saved by each of you based on the salaries. It'll get you into a mode of doing something special together. You will also share the comfort of knowing that both of you are equally invested in creating something so beautiful and special for yourselves.

Your working would be as follows:

Total Pre-pregnancy cost (X) = prenatal care + delivery cost

Number of months before you start trying to conceive (N)

Amount to be saved per month (M) = X/N

Amount to be saved by each of, if equal (E) = M/2

Please also bear in mind that if you are salaried, your employer's Mediclaim policy might just cover pregnancy costs. You might feel awkward about going to HR and asking about it way before you are expecting. Instead, try asking your colleagues with kids what they know about it. If the Mediclaim does cover pregnancy and ancillary costs, get a list of the same. Some larger companies also have a list of pre-approved medical practitioners or hospital chains with whom they would prefer to deal. Often even insurance companies have specifications about what qualifies for a claim and what doesn't. It would be good for you if you could make sure you know where to go and with whom to deal in order to get your claim easily.

A good practice would be to make a file and put every bill and document related to the pregnancy process in it. This includes the Mediclaim policy copy, the list of agencies approved by the insurer, medical reports, prescriptions, and all bills from the pathology labs and doctors' visits. This may sound pretty paranoid, but filing reports and stuff is handy whenever you need to visit the doctor. Believe me, you are not being paranoid. When you start your regular visits, the first thing they'll ask you for at the hospital reception will be your file. Bigger hospitals also have patient unique ID numbers to help locate your electronic records. Like me, if you don't remember your patient ID, you can provide the registered mobile number.

For those who may not be aware, one of the biggest advantages of going with the approved institutions of the insurer is that you can go cashless. That means that you don't need to pay the delivery bills first and then claim the refund. You can submit the list of documents asked by the hospital and have the insurance company pay the hospital directly. Your money doesn't get blocked till the claim comes through and there's hardly any stress for you at all.

We live in an age where people don't ask enough of the right questions. Either they're too shy or scared to ask the relevant questions or they couldn't care less. That attitude is the downfall of our species today. Because we don't want to question what we know to be wrong or don't take the trouble to be well-informed, we waste precious resources and end up spending unnecessary amounts of money.

Make it a habit to ask your doctors and the hospitals whether every item you are being asked to pay for, whether a test or medicine, is necessary and why. If you know why it's required, you don't mind paying for it, but if it's being dumped on you without good reason, why not question it? Even if it's covered by insurance, the insurance company may be paying for something unnecessary. So make it a habit to go through the bills and ask why.

When I was getting discharged from the hospital after my second kid, we realised that the bill had a bottle of enema medication and 3 packs of diapers billed to us. I had never been given an enema, before or after the delivery. And over a 2 and a half day stay at the hospital, we had only consumed about 14 diapers. Definitely not 3 packs. We managed to get those costs reduced, and though the amounts are not much, it's a case in point.

A small disclaimer here, though. Information is power, but half-baked information can lead to disaster. In the age of the internet and Google, we no longer have the patience to wait to hear what the doctor has to say. We google our symptoms and find answers from thousands of websites and blogs that claim to be experts. However, at the end of each of these, they will always tell you that you should seek professional advice if the problem persists. In many situations, we take the partial information that we get from these sources to our doctors and end up arguing with them based on it. My doctor has a little plaque outside her cabin that says, "Please do not confuse your Google search with my medical degree!"

What I'm saying is that although you must be alert and not trust blindly, use your judgement carefully. Let your discretion be led by your trust and let your questions be based on the desire to gain more knowledge, not the need to prove your doctor wrong. When you ask questions of someone who is an expert in their domain, if you are humble in your approach, it makes for a constructive conversation. If you try to show off that you can't be taken for a ride, you might just end up irritating someone who is being perfectly reasonable and has your best interests in mind.

Plan well, stay ahead of the curve. The meter of your bill starts from the moment you start thinking of having the baby.

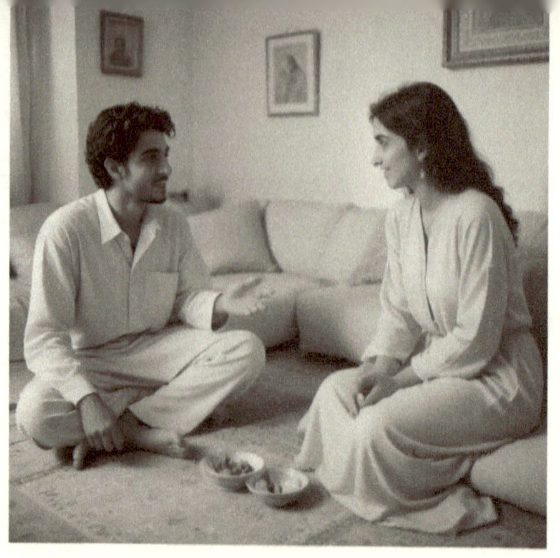

Chapter 11

PROBLEMS IN CONCEPTION

Varun and Sonal got married in their early 30s. They met through a common friend and hit it off. They were both looking to settle down and found each other compatible. They each met the other's major preferences in a potential partner and wanted similar things at that point in life. Just the year before their marriage, Varun had started a new business and was working really hard to set it up. Sonal had a well-paying job and really loved her work. In the middle of all that, a baby was not a priority. It wasn't until after Sonal's younger sister had a kid and they both realised that they were in their last 30s that the swift passage of time hit them. It was also around that time that their business had really taken off and Sonal quit her job to help Varun out. They also started trying for a baby.

Things were good on one front, they weren't so great on another. Having a baby wasn't easy. Not only were both of them approaching 40, but they were also both unfit and had various health issues like high cholesterol, borderline diabetes, and hypertension. It was not only about getting pregnant but also about being mentally and physically healthy to raise the child. They tried a lot of things before their doctor finally suggested IVF (in vitro fertilisation). Sonal got pregnant in her fourth IVF cycle. Going through the process was really a struggle as IVF requires a lot of medication and injections. It also took immense mental fortitude to try another round after each unsuccessful attempt. But they kept at it. Maybe it was the stories of others who had seen success after multiple attempts or their own burning desire for a child, but they did keep trying. Their son's birth was no less than a hard-earned miracle for them.

Varun and Sonal aren't the only ones. Millions of people are going through problems related to conception that are in part natural and in part man-made. The shape of the woman's uterus, blocked fallopian tubes, lazy ovaries. These things and more can cause problems in having a baby in an otherwise perfectly healthy woman and will need medical intervention.

While the problems related to female infertility may often be identified long before the couple starts trying to conceive, male infertility is usually identified, if at all, only after the couple has been trying persistently for a while. This is because female infertility problems could also cause irregular periods or other symptoms in women which are often identified and treated by the women out of concern for their overall well-being. Except cases of delayed ejaculation or suspected lack of potency, it is unlikely that anyone would suspect male infertility. There is treatment for the various causes of male infertility as well, depending upon the underlying problem.

Usually, doctors advise every couple to first try normally. The window would be about 2 years in a reasonably healthy and young couple and up to a year in a couple that is slightly older. If even then things don't work out, the doctor would want to investigate the causes. The procedure would involve some blood tests to check for things like iron deficiency, blood sugar, or hyperthyroidism and some scans to help identify any physiological anomaly. The results will help the doctor determine whether or not there is a problem that requires treatment. Sometimes the problem may be rectified through a simple change in habits or a bit of medication and sometimes, more complex help may be required.

High school biology tells us about the complex machinery of the human body. It has various smaller systems that perform critical functions – the respiratory system, the digestive system, the nervous system and so on. The reproductive system is the one that draws the most giggles and sniggers in any biology class. It's also one that can cause havoc in your nervous system when you progress in life.

After my miscarriage, I really beat myself up. I kept asking myself why I had gone to Ladakh, why did I have to go for that party the night before I did the test and why I had not taken better care of my health through the years. Surely the fault must be with me. As I realised with time, there was no fault to be laid with me. I had actually conceived during that trip and it wasn't planned. I had gone for the party with family and did the test on impulse although my period wasn't even due (yes, it was instinct that drove me to do the test). I was quite fit and although a little overweight, there was nothing medically wrong with me. That baby was just not meant to be.

The foetus would have to be analysed in a lab to understand why it had stopped growing after 6 weeks and even then, there might not be an answer. My doctor very patiently explained that such miscarriages are fairly common and really not the fault of anyone. Sometimes, if the particular egg or sperm that have mated are not healthy enough, the foetus is also unhealthy and won't grow. Sometimes, the foetus doesn't get connected to the wall of the uterus properly and that can also lead to problems. None of these are things in anyone's control.

Conception is a tricky process and any number of things can be the reason behind it not working out when you want.

Also, difficulty in conception doesn't necessarily mean you're infertile. It could be an absolute stroke of fate or a matter of wrong timing or simply a result of bad habits. But fear not. Most of these problems have some kind of remedy in modern medicine. Let's get the serious dough on it through our expert writer.

Expert Speak

How many people are needed to make a baby? Two: of course, yes. What does it take to make a baby? Generally, it needs a couple who can have sex. If the act occurs when the woman is in her fertile phase and one of the millions of sperms that have been released in the vagina is able to swim up the uterus and fallopian tube and mate with an egg that has been released: voila! You have a pregnancy.

If achieving a pregnancy is so easy, why then do some couples make such heavy weather? Multiple factors may be responsible. First and foremost, even if a normal couple has sex in the fertile period, the chances of conceiving are hardly 15-16% in any given cycle. Therefore, doctors ask couples to try for a pregnancy naturally for a year before doing all the evaluation and investigations for infertility. In older couples, the waiting period is reduced to 6 months.

The woman needs to be in good general health. Chronic conditions such as diabetes, thyroid dysfunction, and high blood pressure need to be brought under control. The woman is evaluated for ovulation (development and release of an egg). Generally, sonography is done on a serial basis to ensure that a follicle is developing in the ovary and that the egg or oocyte is being released properly. Once the egg is released from the ovary, it has to be transported into the fallopian tube, where fertilisation occurs. Thus, in women who do not conceive, the doctor performs tests that check the patency of the tubes. These tests may be done with the help of an X-ray machine (hysterosalpingogram), an ultrasound machine (sonosalpingography), or the tubes may be checked at the time of surgery (chromopertubation at laparoscopy). The uterus and its lining are evaluated by ultrasound since that is where the pregnancy grows. If there is any local infection in the vagina, it is treated with locally applied or orally ingested medications.

The male partner will invariably be asked to get his semen sample evaluated. The sample is collected by masturbation, after 3 days' abstinence from either sex or masturbation. The man's semen sample may be fine but his performance may not. Thus, he is asked about impotence or premature ejaculation and treated as the case may be.

The Male Factor

It takes 2 to make a child. Though in India, the whole family feels that they should be an integral part of the process as well. This puts a lot of pressure on the poor male, not just on the woman. To the extent that men complain of an inability to perform: it may be difficult to get an erection and sometimes having achieved an erection, it may be difficult to sustain the erection or to achieve ejaculation. Problems with erection and ejaculation may need evaluation and treatment with medications.

One of the standard evaluations done in a male is the evaluation of his semen. This helps detect problems like low sperm count and low sperm motility (i.e., the ability of the sperm to swim ahead). In other cases, there may be abnormal forms of sperm which means that the head or tail of the sperm is misshapen. Although a misshapen sperm may still be able to fertilise an egg, a high number of abnormal sperms may cause male infertility. This can be treated in most cases with medication and lifestyle changes.

In the case of some men, the semen may be viscid or sticky. This also can lead to poor fertility. If testing of the sperm sample shows the presence of pus cells in the semen, it signifies an infection in the semen and would require treatment with antibiotics.

Improving one's lifestyle, reducing stress, avoiding excessive alcohol and tobacco consumption go a long way in improving male fertility. It has been observed that overheating of the scrotum and testes due to the use of tight underwear or working in high-temperature environments such as furnace areas also leads to issues with male fertility. This just goes to show that the human body, whether male or female, though highly resilient, is very sensitive and requires to be looked after well.

For most of the above problems, a proper course of multivitamins containing zinc and co-enzymes will help. If the count and motility are still low after treatment, the couple can opt for more advanced procedures to aid conception.

The human body is incredibly resilient and strong. The kind of pain a woman endures to bring out the baby is testimony to that. When the delivery is through caesarean section, the surgeon cuts through 7 layers of body tissue to get the baby out; yes, 7 layers. Women heal enough within a few days to not only carry on with their routine lives but also raise their newborn child. You have to have faith in your ability to be that person who can not only have the child but also go through the trials and tribulations it may take to get you there. Don't lose hope. Hang in there. It may not happen when you expected it to but it will happen when it must. After all, every child that is born has his or her destiny preordained.

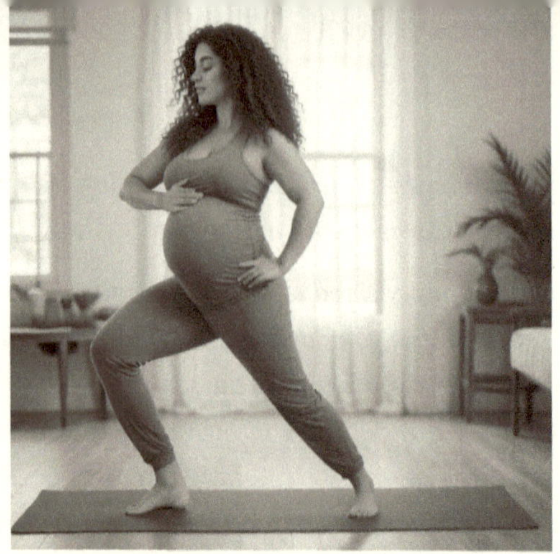

Chapter 12

PHYSICAL FITNESS AND PREGNANCY

Komal and Pradeep live in an upmarket locality of Bangalore. They had been married for 6 years when they conceived. It was an assisted conception that resulted in twins, one boy and one girl. Komal had been quite skinny for most of her life, and she would never have imagined in her 20s that she would have trouble conceiving at all. However, the lifestyle and carelessness towards her own body added up. She didn't know until she started trying to conceive that she had thyroid issues. Within a couple of years, she had gained 20 kilos. While initially, people told her that the extra weight looked good on her, once she crossed a certain line, friends started asking her about it. By then, they had been trying naturally for a baby for about a year. It was only when they visited a gynaecologist that she was asked to get her thyroid tested.

It's not that she was struggling to conceive because of the thyroid or something, but the thyroid-induced weight gain and the hormonal changes that came with a stressful routine did have something to do with it. As the years passed and the problem went unaddressed, the need for remedial action grew. The doctor advised her that she could start yoga and meditation and wait a few months until her hormones were back under control, but she wasn't willing to. The years were ticking by, and she didn't want to compromise on her career either. This was the right time, in her opinion.

It's wrong to judge Komal for her choices; any of us could be in the same boat and making the same or worse choices. But what you can do is see what could have been done better.

The worst thing about youth is that when you have it, you don't value it. We don't really appreciate that when we are old, our bodies will also age or that we will become vulnerable at some point in time. And this is perhaps why we don't take good care of ourselves and our bodies when we have the time and ability to do it. Whether or not you are about to get pregnant, irrespective of your sex and age, you should consider fitness a top priority. All of us should. More so if you're planning on bringing the monumental responsibility of a child into your life. If you want to be able to give the best of yourself to your baby, don't you think you owe it to your child to take good care of yourself?

Becoming healthy doesn't mean just being slim or a certain weight. You could have an hourglass figure or weigh exactly as per the charts for your height and still not only be unfit but also suffer from any number of conditions that you didn't know of. Diabetes, hypertension, anaemia, thyroid, and cholesterol are some of the most common ones that take root without us realising it.

Our definition of healthy has been conditioned to mean good-looking. Living in the age of Instagram and Facebook hasn't helped matters either. The beauty of our photos is far more important than the health of the bodies underlying them. They're not the same thing. Someone who is healthy probably looks good, but just because someone fits into a certain size of clothes, doesn't mean they're healthy.

When you decide to become a parent, you should start taking your lifestyle and fitness more seriously than before. It is not something that has to start only once you know the baby is on its way. It would be ideal to be conscious of your health from an early age. But if you haven't taken care always, you should at least switch gears from the day you set your mind to wanting to be a parent. That could be 2 years or 10 years before, but it has to start then. It's because how you live your life now that decides what kind of body and mind you have by the time you actually become a parent. Unlike the age of the baby boomers when people were having babies around 25-21 years of age, in our times, most suburban fathers are over 30 years old, while most mothers are over 27 years old. That means that the average age by which you will send your children off to college would definitely be over 45 years for both of you.

If most of us want to retire around 60, by 30 years of age we are halfway through our working life. At 45-40, we are at the peak of our lives, when we've established ourselves and have a lot of the struggles sorted. The years that will require you to physically spend yourself in caring for your child are in this phase, where your body is past its prime. These are also the years when you take up a lot of mental stress because you are riddled with responsibility and your body is no longer what it used to be. Growing children and ageing parents are a very difficult combination but one that we must all deal with. Therefore, it's imperative that you stay physically and mentally fit longer than your parents since you will be much older when your kids are growing up.

We don't start ailing from any of the lifestyle-related diseases overnight. We develop them over a period of time as a result of bad habits and/or genetics. It takes years of wear and tear to make a resilient organism like the human body deteriorate to a level where a certain part of it doesn't function at the optimum level. For example, diabetes is a condition of the pancreas, and you don't get diabetes overnight. It takes years of neglect or bad habits to lead you there. I'm sure no one thinks of it that way because when you think of diabetes, you only think of blood sugar levels.

Type 1 diabetes is the result of an autoimmune disease where the insulin-producing cells are destroyed by the body, and so one needs to take injections of insulin to regulate blood sugar. There's no known cure for type 1 diabetes yet. If you're ailing from it, you will need to take extra precautions after discussing with your doctors in order to get pregnant and throughout your pregnancy.

Type 2 diabetes or diabetes mellitus is a different matter. It is the result of poor lifestyle habits, brought on by weight gain, lack of exercise, poor dietary intake, frequent alcohol consumption, or a combination of any of these factors. This is something one can avoid or reverse with changes in lifestyle. It would mean eating right and exercising regularly. For those with more severe problems, medication may also be required. While you may think that you don't really eat out a lot or have healthy habits, you will be surprised to know what a diabetologist or nutritionist think of the food you eat.

We can't assume things. Put in the effort to read and learn about the food you are eating and that which you should actually be eating. Start with reading the labels on your ready-made food purchases. There's a lot of information available on the internet that can help you obtain a better understanding of what your body needs and how it works, without breaking the bank. Better to spend on good quality foods and nutrition than on medicines later in life.

There are also lots of apps and support groups on social media that can help you reclaim your body and life. Download an app to help monitor your food intake. You can log in every item of food you consume to know what kind of nutrition has gone into your body and make changes accordingly, at least in terms of macros. Macros mean the content of your food in terms of macronutrition, i.e., proteins, fats, and carbohydrates. Micronutrients mean the vitamin and mineral content of your food. All of these apps will help you track with reasonable accuracy the macros of your food intake. At the same time, you can opt for multivitamin supplements to ensure your micronutrient intake is also up to the mark.

Apart from this, there's a wide array of fitness apps that help you not only monitor how much you've walked on a given day and how many stairs you've climbed but also how many calories you've burned by doing so and how much more you need to do. Get active. Ditch the stairs, make your water bottle your constant companion, and use your phone for more than just responding to mails and texts and watching crappy content. These are all building blocks of a **fitter you**. If you start tracking your nutrition and exercise, chances are that you will end up rectifying the gross negligence that you've subjected your body to easily. If your problems still persist despite consistent focus, you can definitely opt for expert advice.

Stress is another key player in determining how your body tolerates the changes it undergoes. Work-related stress is at an all-time high in the modern world and is one of the major causes of high blood pressure and diabetes. Extended work days and long work hours lead to unhealthy eating, inadequate sleep, and decline in your body's immunity. The longer you persist in the vicious cycle of eat-work-eat-sleep-repeat, the worse it gets. Your mind stops functioning at capacity, your body starts showing signs of wear and tear, and your system starts shutting down. The body is a living machine; it's definitely going to show the wear!

Pregnancy can be a game-changer for you if you want to get off that never-ending cycle we spoke about. Start looking at yourself more closely. Don't let your inertia defeat you. For most people, it's not a question of ability, but only a question of the will to get in shape. My own gym trainer from my days before marriage was a fitness freak married to a foodie. His wife couldn't care less about what she ate or whether she worked out. He had been trying to convince her to change her habits for years without success. Eventually, when they started trying for a baby, they struggled to conceive. She was told by the doctor to shed some weight before she could be put on some of the medications as they led to weight gain. That became a turning point for her. Eventually, not only did she become fitter but also became a fitness trainer like her husband. She's one of my greatest inspirations of what a person can do if they want to.

Are you beginning to wonder why you have to sacrifice so much for the sake of a child? Please remember that these changes to your lifestyle are for your personal betterment. They will ensure you are at your optimum performance levels, physically and mentally. If you do improve your health, not only will your chances of having a baby and ability to cope with child-rearing improve, your overall appearance and your professional life will also benefit. Leading a healthy life will aid your professional growth as well because your mind will become sharper, and your overall ability to deal with problems will improve. If it feels like too much effort, keep reminding yourself that you are doing it all firstly for yourself.

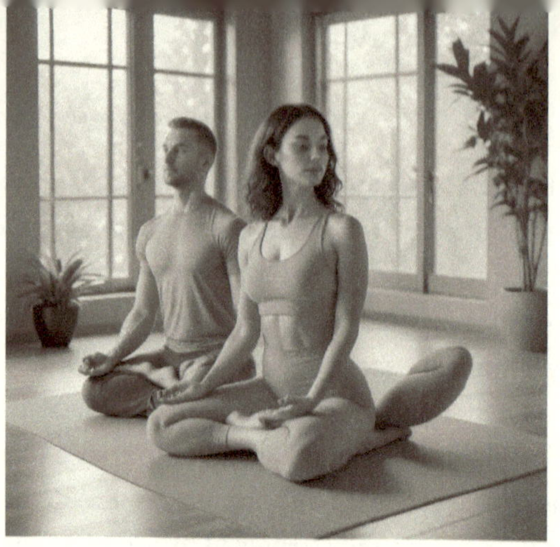

<h2 style="text-align:center">Chapter 13</h2>

PHYSICAL FITNESS FOR THE OTHER PARENT

Sujay and Kirti fit the profile of the quintessential educated, woke couple who believe they have to give back more to society than they have received. They are equals in everything – they both partake of household duties and are employed by blue-chip firms. Both have excellent careers and a wonderful family life. When their older daughter was born, Sujay took his paternity leave to help care for their daughter. He did what he could for her on a daily basis – baths, diaper changes, walks in the park, and meals. So, the decision to have another child was not difficult for Kirti. But around the time of the birth of their second child, Sujay started having back problems. He had been an athlete during his school and college days but after joining a corporate, his lifestyle had obviously changed. While he was still reasonably fit on medical parameters, his body was definitely worse for the wear. As a result, he couldn't really help Kirti with the younger one, and even helping out with the older child was only possible to a certain extent and excluded any kind of serious physical strain.

Sujay's story is not one-off. Given that fewer men take the time out for their own fitness in a world that is hell-bent on a rat race, being physically fit is becoming a challenge for many men, even at a young age. Add to that the general attitude of mard ko dard nahi hota and you have people completely ignoring their health. It's not until the multiple daily pills start and the doctor strongly advises exercise or in some cases even physiotherapy that people realise the fault with this mindset.

If raising a child was just one person's job, we wouldn't be having this discussion. All families are different. Some have grandparents, some don't. Some have both parents, some have 2 moms, and some have one. Whichever kind of family yours happens to be, one thing is certain – if you want a child, then you are a parent. If you are a parent, you will have responsibilities. The role of a parent doesn't start and finish at childbirth. But since there is so much focus on this one part of the process in the beginning of the journey, not enough is said about the role of the other parent and there is no focus on the health or fitness of that person. This is wrong and unfair. For a lot of reasons.

The need to be fit is not applicable only to the women who want to conceive. The need to be physically fit applies equally to the other parent. As soon as one partner conceives or there is talk of a baby in the house, the lives of both people are about to change drastically. The need for each of you to be fit is as high because both of you are going to be part of the process of raising the child. You may not realise it now, but both of you will have sleepless nights, both of you will spend a lot of time carrying around a baby that grows every single minute, and both of you will feel the pain that the baby goes through. How are you supposed to be able to handle so much more if your body and mind are not up to it? No, this is important for both of you.

It's not just about breastfeeding and changing diapers. Once I was pregnant, I wasn't the only one who had extra stuff to do. My husband had to make up for a lot of stuff that was usually on my plate but I was no longer able to do. He was scheduling my tests, driving me to the lab for the sonography, getting me snacks to eat when I was suddenly hungry, lugging my handbag because I was breathless… the list is endless. Not to mention putting up with my hormone-induced mood swings, unstoppable midnight cravings, and meltdowns brought about by my fears and anxieties.

There were days when I would be upset about my old clothes no longer fitting me. I have said this often – why do I alone have to get fat if we're both having the baby! What is any husband or partner supposed to say to a statement like that?!!!! There's no answer, let alone there being a perfect one. Putting up with a demanding, self-assured woman who's going through the travails of pregnancy can really fray the nerves of anyone. So being fit at least physically is a bare minimum if you have to cope with all that extra stress. And it's not like your regular, mundane responsibilities are going anywhere to make room for the new ones.

The mother-to-be is going to increasingly find it difficult to meet her obligations. As the pregnancy progresses, she will tire easily and will need help with more and more things. Not only will her body suffer but her mind will also make it hard for her to cope with the pressures of life that she was earlier a pro at handling. Hormones tend to play truant and make women highly emotional during a pregnancy. They tend to cry at the drop of a hat and are pretty likely to start fighting over rather petty matters. So, you need to up your game to make up for all that friction and keep some semblance of sanity going in your home.

Late nights are eventually not for the mother alone either. You would want to be there for your child and help soothe her in the toughest moments. That means lesser sleep for extended time periods. Also, the bigger family means more expenses. You can't afford to let go of your job or compromise on your work. To the contrary, we tend to get into this happy high that drives us to give our best to everything so that we can give the best to our children. All of this adds more pressure on your body, right? Getting fit is as relevant to being a good parent as being well-informed, educated or emotionally available.

An unfit body and a tired mind aren't recipes for successful people. Having a baby often sets the mother back in her career, and if she opts to continue to work at the same pace as before because her husband is actively pitching in, then it's possible that even the father will suffer in his career. If you don't want that to happen, you need to train yourselves to cope with 2 full-time jobs, not just one. Your old one pays in cash and your new one pays in love. You can't make a choice between the 2, and honestly, if you're reading this book, I can tell that you don't want to make one.

One of the things my husband has enjoyed during his days as a father is a lot of extra attention. I'm serious. Just because I was busy didn't mean he wasn't getting attention. He was getting it from all the women he met at the park while taking my little one for a stroll in her gleaming new pram! One of his most favourite things to do over a period of time became to take our daughter there because not only did he get to work out in the process but he would often be approached by women who were admiring the baby. As per his own assessment, they were admiring the handsome and hands-on father as well! While this will be easy for any parent to implement after the baby arrives, you need to build the habit from now, right?

Start cutting down on the vices – overeating, smoking, drinking, not sleeping enough over Netflix or WhatsApp, late nights at work. These things don't do anyone a favour, and there's a time in life when every excess has to be corrected. If you don't make the effort to do it while you have a say in the matter, soon there will be a day when you don't necessarily have a choice. If you control your food intake and lead a disciplined life, you will be able to get away with the odd bingeing once in a while and not be any worse off.

Start trading your normal practices for healthier ones. Ditch the elevator, walk while you take a long call, cut down on sugar, avoid fried food, and make sure to have some fruit every day. One other thing that our elders often tell us but we choose to ignore is caffeine. Tea and coffee, while offering tons of solace, actually have practically no nutritional value and high-calorie content. They're bad for us all, especially if you're like me and find that a cup of tea or coffee is the first thing that comes to mind when thinking or ideating or working or doing nothing at all! I've tried to cut back over the years, but tea made me nauseous during my pregnancies, and I had to avoid it for almost 5 months each time.

I want to stress here the importance of the back. The back is one of the most prone areas for those living in urban cities. Spondylitis, slipped disc, and lower back pain are some of the most common forms of back trouble. These can be caused by excessive sitting, obesity, lack of exercise, and stress. Yoga is the best way to avoid these problems and can go a long way in alleviating any of these conditions if you're already suffering from them. Eventually, you'll have to carry around the baby a lot and also the baby's diaper bag. If you do have recurring back pain, do yourself a favour and tend to it seriously now.

Yoga is extremely popular all over the world for pregnancy and general fitness. In India, we have easy access to yoga classes and teachers, but we don't make enough out of these. Yogasanas are available for almost every known ailment of the body, and regular practice can help you attain not only a fitter body but also a calmer mind. Since it requires so much focus, yoga can really help you reduce your stress levels and take you on the long-term path to health.

Planning ahead to make sure you start changing your lifestyle will help you deal with the pressure of raising a child much better.

If you're smart enough to plan for the monetary expenditure, why not plan for the self-expenditure as well? What do I mean by self-expenditure? It is using yourself to your capacity, whether mentally or physically. Money is fungible and can be replaced, but you are not a replaceable commodity. No one can give that warmth and comfort to your child or the kind of attention the child needs other than you. You need to be at the top of your game as your performance as a parent has to be top-class as well!

In the process of becoming fit, both of you could try to work as a team. Motivate each other to be better versions of yourselves. Help each other deal with your weak areas. Become a source of encouragement and inspiration, not destructive criticism. I've been guilty of that by nature, but I've worked on it and have monitored my husband's health as much as I have my own. It's been years of work to get someone who hates the idea of doodhi or turai to eat vegetables other than potato. Believe me, it does take time to break old habits and help people develop new ones. A smaller thing like your partner taking 2 spoons of sugar in one glass of milk may not seem important right now, but when you put things in perspective, it does need correction. It would be a lot easier if you worked on it together and knowing well that there was an added reason for it – your baby.

But alas, are you doing this just for your baby? No. You must do this as much for each other and yourself. Being fit increases your ability to support your partner. It increases *your self-confidence* and helps you be better at the things you do. It will all pay in the form of increased stamina and greater endurance. These, in turn, will help you deal with the curveballs that life throws at you unexpectedly. So please, remember that the whole garden matters, not just one plant.

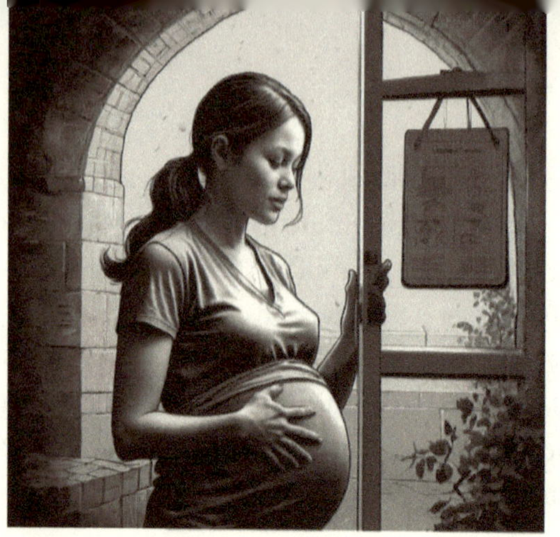

Chapter 14

THE EMOTIONAL BURDEN OF WANTING TO GET PREGNANT

Nisha always knew she wanted to be a mother. Right from playing baby-baby with her dolls, to volunteering to be the one to monitor her younger cousins, to getting a part-time job during college at a daycare centre to finally making sure she married someone who wanted to have a family, it was always a large part of who she was going to be in life eventually. The same goes for another friend of mine, Manish. Even when Manish was visiting cousins, friends, or colleagues, he was the one who would soon be found entertaining the children or the one to whom the children would naturally gravitate if there was a fight or someone got hurt. He never turned them down and found it easy to bring a smile to their faces. When both of these people eventually decided to start a family with their respective partners, there was a lot of intensity going into the whole thing. The underlying desire was very strong and it wasn't okay to not have a baby.

Nisha had a good career going for her. She was so particular about wanting a baby by a certain age that she quit her job and started doing freelance assignments so that she could free up time for the pregnancy and baby whenever it happened. The decision to quit wasn't a good one for many reasons. Not only did it mean that she had more time to focus on her pregnancy, but it also meant that she had more time to worry about it not happening soon. Instead of living her normal life and going through the process like most others do, she was so focused on it that she spent a lot of time every day planning out her personal life as per her ovulation cycle. If you talk to any doctor, they will tell you that this is the last thing you should do if you want to conceive easily. So much focus and stress are not going to help your hormones, and the changes in life and lifestyle will only add to your woes.

After living this life for 2 years, Nisha and her husband decided to finally see a doctor who told them that she had blocked fallopian tubes. She had literally wasted 2 years of her working life. Although she did conceive eventually and is now a happy mother, she cannot deny that the stress she went through because of the choices she made around her desire to have a baby by the date set in her own mind could have been avoided. Her career has never really recovered, but since the baby was so important to her, fortunately, she doesn't regret it much. What she does regret though is the excess focus she put into the whole thing which not only deprived her of peace of mind for almost 2 years but also put strain on her relationship with her husband. His practical approach to the matter against her almost obsessive focus led to many avoidable arguments and fights. The cycle of try-test-cry-repeat can be so stressful for both parties that it can literally ruin half of your days every month.

We go through school and spend most of our adulthood being told that the most important organ in our bodies is our brain. We spend so much time trying to improve its functioning and the kind of content we put into it, that we do little else until we pass the threshold of adulthood. There is constant focus on 'learning better, learning more, learning the right thing.' But there is no learning for strengthening our resolve or building patience for the bigger challenges of life.

The heart is the centre of a lot of the poetry in this world, but not enough is said about learning for the heart. It is projected as a vault for either our feelings or all the cholesterol in the world. As if our feelings are something we should be ashamed of or something we should hide. There are no coaching classes to teach us how to cope with the innumerable feelings we deal with, sometimes so many of them clouding our hearts and minds at the same time. We are overwhelmed by them at times when things are completely out of our control. One of the most vulnerable such times in our lives is when we are getting onto the rollercoaster of parenting.

From the very day you figure out that you want to have a baby, you start feeling a sense of anticipation. Anticipation of what it would be like to have a kid of your own, when you will be able to have the baby, whether it will be easy or difficult, will it happen quickly or you'll have to keep trying forever, whether you'll make a good parent, whether your partner will be able to support you the way you expect them to through it all, whom the child will look like......... the list is quite endless.

Once you've started trying for a baby, the stress and the emotional pressure are unbelievable. Every month, you start counting days. First to your ovulation window and then to your period date. Each time, there's a clock ticking in your mind as you first wait for your period and if it's even a day late, you rush to do the home test. You can't bear to wait. Every cycle, you hope that your miracle will come through but it doesn't work out that easily. And the wait, it really chips away at you, one day at a time.

If you've gone through a few cycles and been disappointed, the tears start coming. You begin to question what you did wrong or why the hell you deserve this. You start feeling like you would make a better parent than most people you know and have never indulged in any stupid vices, so why are you getting punished? If your partner doesn't share your anxiety and excitement, you start resenting them for going about their life normally whilst you are in tatters! You hate them for not sharing your feelings. On the contrary, if your partner does keep track of things and is as eager as you to get pregnant, then every time they ask you how many days to go or they stock up on the test kit, you'll most likely get really pissed off! It's not a good phase to go through.

A friend of mine went through almost 6 IUI cycles to have her second daughter. She was really desperate the second time as her older child was already 9 years old by then. The physical and mental pain she went through trying to have her second one took a terrible toll on her body which was by default not completely fit. Eventually, she got her menopause impossibly early (it started by the time she was 37) and along with it came a mild form of arthritis which flares up for no reason at all. I know how hard it is for her to cope with regular tasks on days when the arthritis is particularly bad and sometimes makes me wonder whether it was really worth it. In hindsight, she didn't know this would happen. She had only been trying to follow her heart and gone after what she really, really wanted!

When you start trying for a child, sometimes, you don't care what cost it comes at. It really does consume everything you are – your personal life, your career, your sensibilities, everything. You tend to start ignoring everything else. You become part of a race which doesn't exist anywhere except in your own mind. Your mental health takes a huge beating under the burden of this desire and desperation. This also affects your body because stress will definitely play havoc with your hormones. The tears, the anger, the resentment, it all comes with a price.

Unbeknownst to you, your partner's state of mind is also suffering. You become unavailable to them and expect them to be there with you for the ride. They do share in your pain and disappointment, maybe not always to the extent you want but they are part of the journey with you, isn't it? You are here, trying for the child, because BOTH of you want it. Unlike you, maybe your partner isn't in a tearing rush and maybe they believe that it will happen when it has to. Don't beat them up about it.

No, you don't do any of this consciously, but it's a terrible thing that does happen. You become sort of like Gollum from Lord Of The Rings, maniacal in your desire and your longing. None of this is healthy for your relationship. You have gotten to the stage of trying after making a lot of decisions TOGETHER. There is a value attached to that. Don't write that off. Respect your partner's needs as you expect them to respect yours. Give them space because not everyone deals with emotions like you do. I learnt this the hard way too. I couldn't understand why my husband seemed fine after my first miscarriage while I was going through so much. It wasn't his fault. We hadn't planned the baby and though he was as thrilled about it as I was at the time, he didn't feel like the earth had come crashing down just because it hadn't worked out. Today, I realise how unfair my assessment of his attitude as cavalier and callous was. He just didn't feel like it was such a big deal. It wasn't his fault that I did!

If you are going through so much turmoil, talk to the people you are close to. Don't shut them off. The prenatal state of mind needs to be cared for properly. How are you going to get through your pregnancy and parenthood eventually if you crumble from now itself? Don't lose heart and start considering yourself weak. Build your resilience and prepare yourself to handle these things. Get the help you need, whether from family, friends or maybe even a professional.

Incidentally, this process teaches you a thing or 2 about yourself and others as well. If someone you know, who's on the same life trajectory as you, conceives before you, you'll realise you're not the nice person you thought you were. You'll feel envy and hatred of a kind that you never knew you were capable of. You'll end up spending a few thousand hours trying to figure out what they did different from you and why the hell are they pregnant when you aren't! Even if that someone is your own sibling or best friend, you'll feel resentment about them getting ahead in this so-called race. It may seem impossible right now, but you'll realise it's not that easy to feel happy for others when you're in your own little rut!

It gets worse. You also start judging people. Anyone who tries to calm you down and says, "Don't worry. It'll happen when it has to," is an enemy and an idiot of the topmost degree! What do they know of your pain and anxiety, and how are they supposed to understand what you feel when they've never been through what you're going through?! Yeah. It'll happen. My own mother has been in that position. I've actually told mom at one point that she would never know what it felt like to be me because she had kids at 23-22 and had managed to conceive both of us within a year of each other! Today, we can sit back and laugh about it, but I must admit, I am ashamed of having taken out my frustration on her. She, of course, being the generous mother she is, took it in her stride and just let me vent!

The anger becomes a constant companion. You start losing it at your partner for every suggestion to take it easy for a little while. You start losing it at them for finding someone's baby cute or for congratulating someone else on their pregnancy. You start losing it with them for hell, just saying something completely irrelevant. I mean, how dare they lose focus, right?

It's amazing what the desire for a child can do to a person. It's nothing like greed for money or your ambition for your career. It's the kind of animal desire that no one can explain to you and the kind of longing that only someone who's felt it can understand.

I hear you. I've been through it all. It's unfair and it's unpleasant, but it's perfectly human. It's a call for love. Love because you want someone to love and someone who will always love you. Acknowledge your reality and the emotions but don't let them stampede over your sensitivity to the needs of those around you. Not everyone has reason enough to put up with you. Try and be at least a little considerate of those who are putting up with you because they care. We can often be nastiest to the ones who truly love us. Just because they care doesn't mean we should make them our punching bags!

What will act as fuel to your raging fire is anyone asking you when you're going to plan for a baby. These are people who are really concerned about our biological clock and the state of our marriage. How they feel they're entitled to have an opinion about any of this is beyond my understanding as well, but you can't stop them. People will talk. Ignore what you can't change. Avoid toxic people who don't help your state of mind and try to protect yourself as best as you can by following your normal routine. Normalcy is actually a panacea. It can help us deal with most problems that come out of the blue and keep us steady through storms. Don't stop doing what's normal for you, be it going to work, heading to the gym, taking your annual vacation, or hanging out with your friends.

You're also very likely to become something of a loner in the process of trying to have a baby. Not only will you sometimes alienate yourself from perfectly nice people because they are unable to empathise with you, but you'll also start avoiding being with people just because it makes you feel like a failure or something. That some of your friends already have a kid or that they're pregnant before you or that they're not interested in having a kid, unlike you, will be enough reason for you to want to avoid them. Just because your mother or mother-in-law keeps talking about how wonderful it would be to have a kid in the family, you won't want to talk to them either. Sometimes, you will avoid people only because you want to revel in your misery. The dark confines of your loneliness will feel like a better place than any place where normalcy thrives.

Don't do it. Pull yourself out of this hellhole that you've dug yourself into. Having a child is a normal thing and so is not being able to have the baby on the date you decided you wanted one! Not everyone can get pregnant on the first attempt. Most people will not tell you of their struggles until way after it's over. I remember this crude joke one of my CA lecturers used to make. He used to say that trying to pass CA is like getting pregnant. You never ask how many attempts it took! I realised much later in life how much truth there was to this ridiculous analogy.

The birth of a child is not something one can control. If you have any faith in a greater being, comfort yourself in the knowledge that the birth and death of a person are preordained and determined to happen only when it has to. While you must go through the motions and do whatever your doctors and elders say, don't expect it to happen in a timeframe determined by you. Sometimes, the things we run too hard after elude us the most!

A practical, more reasonable approach towards pregnancy will help relax your body and mind. It will allow your hormones to work better and allow the conscious you to accept help more constructively. You will not find fault where there is none, and your life on the whole will become more liveable. I know it's easier said than done, but once you convince yourself that yes, it will happen when it has to, the emotions become more manageable and the ride less bumpy.

Having a baby is creating a source of and a destination for love. Raising a child is the process of expressing that love and tests its endurance because you will have days when you will wonder why on earth you were so eager to have a monster of your own. It will all pan out, and even then, you will question the sanity of your decisions, more than once. Don't end up pushing away those who love you in the quest for something you don't have. Don't hurt people around you to vent your pain; it doesn't go away like that. The only answer to darkness is light, not more darkness.

Patience is the most important ingredient in the recipe for happiness. Each and every one of us can have a family, to love, nurture, and protect. It doesn't have to be in the way we envisaged it to happen but have faith, you will have a family if you want one. It may not happen when and how you wanted it to, but if you really want it, it will be. Hang in there.

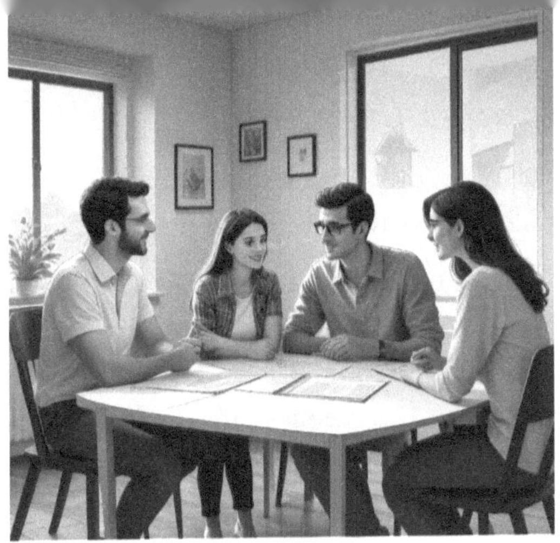

Chapter 15

HOW TO DEAL WITH THE IRRITANTS

Preeti and Palak are identical twins. They've grown up with all the funny and strange tales of the kind of mischief that identical twins get up to because they can easily pass off for each other. Even when they got married, their husbands made them promise not to play pranks involving taking each other's place because it was something they really revelled in. A few years later, Palak conceived her older child. Whenever they were both out together or visiting their parents, people would accidentally ask Preeti how she was doing and when she was due. At first, Preeti didn't mind it but as the days wore on and her own frustration at not having conceived grew, Preeti started getting upset. It got to a level where she started avoiding having to visit her parents' place until Palak's stomach started showing enough for people to know which sister was which. Even then it didn't help because people actually just glancing at her tummy to see which of the 2 sisters she was, made her uncomfortable. It wasn't a pleasant phase of her life and one that she prefers not to talk about.

You can't blame the people around. They don't understand what you're dealing with and how things are going. They have advice, completely unsolicited and totally unwanted, to give for anything and everything; be it someone's life, their relationship status, their pregnancy or children! It's not that these people believe they are perfect or anything. But because they feel they have the best intentions, they dish out soliloquies on the rights and wrongs of life by the second. You have to just assume or accept that they mean well and either listen patiently or ignore. They don't know what you're going through and even if they do, they feel that their bona fide intentions give them the right to say what they please at your expense.

That's why one thing I had a really hard time dealing with when I was trying to get pregnant was the people around me. Their "well-meaning" enquiries about the status of my uterus were not well-received and made me see red all the time. The miscarriage I had had in my first year of marriage had left me scarred emotionally. Although it wasn't a planned pregnancy and we hadn't wanted a baby so early in our marriage, losing the baby had not been easy, especially on me. When the foetus stopped growing at 6 weeks, it felt like some part of me too had died. At that time, our relatives telling us to try again quickly and not delay it, lest there be some real problems with me, was not just irritating but terribly painful. It felt like they were intent on spooning burning hot pepper onto my wounds!

When we found out we were pregnant, we first went to a well-known gynaecologist referred by a family member. She told me to get a couple of tests done. After seeing those, she told me point-blank that I would need to get a D&C. I didn't even know what a D&C was or what that implied. Even after repeatedly asking her to explain what that meant, I didn't comprehend her adequately. She couldn't have been right, you know? I was young, healthy, and had not done anything wrong to lose the baby. It must be some kind of mistake! But no, there was no mistake. She announced her diagnosis as if she was announcing a flight departure. From there, my day was a blur.

We were both hurt, my husband and I. Suddenly, we had found a desire for a baby where there had been none. It had seemed like God's will and therefore, it felt like God's gift was being taken away from us. We felt instant desperation and desolation. It was all unwarranted and unfair. We were only human.

We decided to seek a second opinion. As a result, I met my future friend and the woman who would go on to not only hold my hand through 3 fruitful pregnancies but also deliver my kids and help me write this book, Dr. Salvi. She helped me calm down. She only said one thing, "It happens." She explained that sometimes, foetuses stop growing for no traceable reason and it doesn't mean that something is wrong with me or that I did something bad. It just meant that it wasn't meant to be for now. In hindsight, not only was she right but she was also the reason I didn't start blaming myself. I didn't heap insane loads of self-loathing onto myself or blame for something that wasn't in my control. It really helped me carry on and gave me faith that it would all get better.

One of the most important things is to have people around who you can relate to. Unlike the first doctor I went to, my second one was the right fit for me. She gave me more time and seemed to share my wavelength despite an almost -25year age difference. Every time I met her, it wasn't like she was giving me a long sermon. Quite to the contrary. She'd simply ask, "Yes, what's up today? Let's see the test results" or simply, "Why have you come today? Routine check-up?" She made me feel what I should've felt – NORMAL. That's what a pregnancy is. It's a natural thing and we should deal with it like we deal with any natural phenomena. But that doesn't happen because we revere the idea of getting pregnant. It is so sacred and such a big deal in our country, that to deal with your pregnancy like any other event in our life is unthinkable!

Which is why it's so important to be able to deal squarely with those people who tend to make your life more difficult through it all. You have to have the common sense, fortitude, and immeasurable patience that it takes to ignore most people who do their best to get on your nerves just through the simple act of being their natural selves. It's definitely easier said than done, but putting in the effort to thicken your skin is instrumental in keeping your blood pressure in check!

If you have people in your environment who stress you out more than others, figure out first whether the stress is your doing or theirs. It's going to be easier to change yourself than changing someone else. How do I do that, you ask? Well, ask yourself if that person is the same with you as they are with others and whether others give them the same amount of importance you do. If the answer is no, then clearly the problem is with the person in question because that person has something against you. If the answer is yes, then obviously the problem lies with your reaction, not with that person's natural disposition. If someone is irritating, interfering, or nasty by nature and is generally the same with everyone, then you would do better to ignore them. If you let them get to you when the others around you successfully ignore them, then you would be better off ignoring such a person.

If this is a person who tends to behave differently with you than they do with others, you may want to address the problem with them. If they won't stop doing whatever it is that affects you, you might have to find ways of avoiding interacting with them. Better to use the ABC of human interaction wherever possible rather than go in for a head-on collision! Avoid/Bypass/Confuse. If it's happening unintentionally, you could try to explain to the person in question what it is that is hurting you but don't expect them to necessarily adapt to your need. If you know having a chat won't help, turn a deaf ear or a blind eye, whatever it takes. This is for people you can't avoid.

Some people you can afford to manage or avoid. For example, your regular help, whom you can replace, or a neighbour or friend whom you can do without meeting. Avoid them. Figure out how to stay out of their way because obviously, they have no reason to stay out of yours. Why get into an argument in the first place? It's easier on your nerves, and everyone's happy. Don't feel bad or selfish about it. This is self-preservation. I know my best friend stopped meeting a common friend of ours who couldn't stop talking about how easily she had conceived both her children every time we all met. If she knew that this girl, herself a dentist, was coming to a get-together, she'd first say yes and then eventually never turn up!

If it's your family members who don't seem to be getting it, make it clear that you don't want to hear anything on the topic. Better to stop that train of conversation than to let it become a point of contention. If it's your partner's family members, let your partner do the talking. Start by letting your partner know what you are dealing with and while you're doing so, please try and be considerate. Tell your partner tactfully that so-and-so person is getting on your nerves and causing you undue stress by bringing up a sensitive topic like this. Let them handle it for you. I'm sure if communicated reasonably, any partner would be up to the task or if they don't want to take a direct approach, they'll help you find a mid-way solution. My husband did this for me by telling his family at one point that we didn't want a kid for another couple of years while we still went about our business. That he had said it so blatantly put a stop to unnecessary discussions and gave me space to breathe.

A lot of times, people will step on your toes by telling you what to do and what not to do. Especially if you've been trying to get pregnant for a while, you'll have people telling you that you should give up your job or not do so much work or stop being so ambitious. Agreed, it's none of their business. But you know what I've learnt after 10 years of marriage – other people's opinion about you is none of your business. It's a free world. You can't stop people from having an opinion about anything, so why bother? Either the people in question matter or they don't. If they matter, try and reason with them. Either they'll be convinced or you'll be convinced. If they don't matter, turn a deaf ear. Any problem can be solved if you break it down into smaller pieces rather than treating it like a Godzilla that needs to be bombed!

If everyone is getting to you, it may be time to take a break. You can consider taking a break from trying to get pregnant, or if you don't want to do that, at least take a holiday. A few days in the sun and sand (or whatever your atmospheric fix is) can do wonders for your soul. It can also help reduce the strain on your partner because rest assured, all this drama is taking its toll on him/her too. You can both do a holiday together or if you've been getting on each other's nerves way too much, a few days apart won't do any harm either. It'll give you some much-needed me-time and allow you both to gain perspective.

My husband's best friend's wife is one of the smartest people when it comes to dealing with such situations. They found it really difficult to get pregnant and had not succeeded even after trying for 3 years. She got so sick of the focus from his rather conservative family on her not getting pregnant that she decided to start a business of her own. Even though her own parents tried to dissuade her as they thought it would become a burden when she eventually got pregnant, she persisted and set up a bakery business. Not only is she running her set-up carefully, but the discipline she instilled in her own life to cope with her work paid off and helped her get fitter. She went from being pleasantly plump to super-fit in a year and became pregnant

18 months after setting up her bakery! Eventually, her father-in-law stepped in and helped her take care of the business during the last stage of her pregnancy and the first couple of months when she couldn't make it to work with the kid.

There are a few things I've found really do help people stay sane through such turbulent times in life. A hobby is one of them. It's something everyone tells us to cultivate but we always ignore. One of the best ways to channelise your pent-up energy and emotions is through some kind of creative pursuit. It could be art, music, dance or even cleaning! I found doodling really helped. I had never taken any art classes but the internet is a wonderful place and gives you tons of options to build your creativity. Make it a habit to do something for yourself on a daily basis. It will help you streamline your thoughts and channelise your feelings. You'll feel better at the end of those few minutes or half an hour, whatever you can spare.

Another thing one should seriously consider is meditation or yoga. I find that every once in a while I'll meet someone who looks more stressed than even I am and that I'm suggesting yoga for them. Over a period of time, I started practising it too and it changed my life. Not just yoga or meditation, any form of physical exercise done regularly can help you cope better with your problems because it gives you the satisfaction of having done something solely for yourself. Something away from everyone and everything. It can become your refuge.

Use your time effectively by breaking it into parts dedicated to various pursuits. Part of your day is committed to your professional responsibilities, some part to your personal commitments, some to your basic care like eating, bathing, sleeping. What's left is hardly a few hours. Make a timetable for yourself so that this remaining time can be used effectively and will contribute to your overall well-being.

Another thing that helps to keep your nerves intact when you're biding time is to focus on the other things you do. If you are working, you would be wise to shift the focus of your conversations to your work so that you don't feel vulnerable. It's easier to centre your attention on your strengths than your struggles. So try and stay positive by looking at the things that are going in your favour and keep your friends and family focused on those too. It will help reduce your anxiety when you are around more people and make these occasions happy for you, rather than stressful.

There's something I really would like to share with you at this juncture. Remember, pregnancy is only one battle; it's not the war. You really may not even know what you're getting into. Once you're pregnant, getting through it is another one. After the delivery, the rest of your life begins. It's not all rosy. You'll really have days when you'll question the sanity of having a kid. You'll miss the uncomplicated life before having had your child and long for some peace, quiet and downtime from a never-ending list of deadlines. So take it easy. Once you get into the parents' club, there's no looking back. You're in it for the long haul and it's better to preserve your battery for the bigger fights to come. If you keep sight of the bigger picture, you'll find it easier to not lose your patience and will be able to enjoy your life as it passes before your eyes!

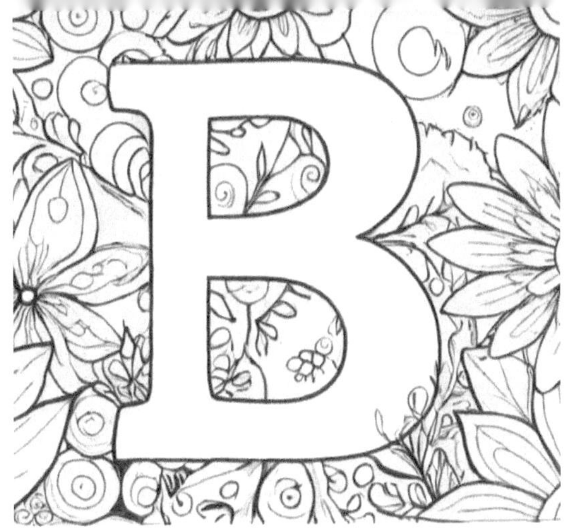

Chapter 16

PLAN B

One of my closest friends, Divya, is an award-winning dancer. She has had the most focused life of all the people I know. Her dance was the most important thing in her life since forever. Her art ensured that not only was she physically fit always but also that she led a well-balanced and reasonably content life. She chased neither money nor success, but her dedication attracted both in abundance. She married her best friend from childhood, and life was beautiful. Until they started trying to have a baby. Divya couldn't conceive despite trying for 2 years. Even after they consulted a doctor, they were told there was no perceptible problem and that they should be patient and keep trying. This went on for another 3 years, and they were really at their wits' end. Finally, after consulting their doctor and family, they opted for assisted reproduction. It worked after the second cycle, and they welcomed a lovely baby after being married for almost 10 years.

What is assisted reproduction? Assisted reproduction is any procedure that involves the handling of the sperm, eggs or both, outside the human body. Basically, any procedure in which the egg or sperm is removed from the human body is called assisted reproduction. Artificial insemination, ovarian stimulation (using medicines), intrauterine insemination (IUI) and in vitro fertilisation (IVF) are all examples of this.

When you started reading this book, I'm not sure which set of people you belong to. You can be one of those who's reading a self-help book way before you set out on the journey. Or you could be someone who's already pregnant and trying to prepare for what's to come. Or you could be someone who's just started trying. Or you could be someone who's struggling with conception. If you belong to the last category, don't lose heart. There's still plenty of time and it can still happen.

There are a lot of options out there. It's not impossible and though it might be a bit expensive and will take longer than you had hoped, it can and will happen. There's tons of scientific stuff happening out there that has changed the way pregnancies happen and how people get through them.

Assisted reproduction is increasingly common. There are a lot of reasons why a bigger number of people are seeking expert help to get pregnant and have a biological child. Although there is no guarantee, most people seeking treatment do get the desired results and sometimes, more! Yes, fertility treatments also often result in multiple babies at a time.

Now don't go cursing yourself or your partner for being in this situation. It's no big deal anymore. Too many people share the same dilemma as you. It's not really something you did to yourself. As we've already discussed in detail, a lot of times, the blame is to be laid on the kind of lifestyles we lead in the modern world and also the quality of nutrition coming from the food we consume.

Since more and more people are pursuing higher education, the incidence of marriage is later in life. Along with that, since both partners are usually working, there is greater stress on their bodies and minds, which results in declined fertility. This is not something one can correct overnight. Just like the problem takes root over a period of time, the solution is also long-term. By the time the knowledge of the problem and the desire to solve it arise, the couple is already feeling behind their planned schedule for life. Therefore, there may be no time to wait to solve the problem at a grassroots level. Hence the need to seek medical aid for conception.

There's a variety of options available to people who have trouble getting pregnant. Depending on the kind of problems you're facing, you will need to seek extra help. Consult your gynaecologist and see whether he/she is equipped to deal with your problem. If they are, then you needn't go anywhere else. If not, they will refer you to a fertility expert or centre. Some solutions are not very intrusive and can help you plan better to aid pregnancy, while other solutions are more intrusive and do put some strain on you. You may have heard complex acronyms like IVF and IUI. We're going to decode some of these here.

Expert Speak

How do we help a couple who are unable to conceive? First, we talk with the couple and ensure that they have no difficulty in having sex on a regular basis. It is not that rare to come across a couple who doesn't know what to do. Or even if they do, they are unable to perform. If they have been trying unsuccessfully, the couple is evaluated further.

The couple is asked whether either smokes, drinks regularly or indulges in any other substance abuse. When it comes to the male, high temperatures are detrimental to fertility. Too hot showers or working in hot environments or excessive heat generation locally as in driving or wearing tight underwear may not be ideal for sperm survival. The male is asked to do his semen evaluation after 3 days of abstinence, but not longer.

If there is any issue, certain medications may be prescribed. Sometimes it may be necessary to get him evaluated by an andrologist for further management.

The woman too needs to be in good general health. For achieving a pregnancy, a few organs need to be in good working order. The ovaries should be producing one egg a month, the tubes should be open to deliver the eggs towards the uterus, the uterus should be normal to support a pregnancy for 9 months, and the vagina should be able to receive sperms that can then actively swim up into the uterus and up the tubes where they can meet and fertilise the egg.

Ovulation, or the act of releasing an egg, is most reliably diagnosed by serial ultrasounds. If the egg is not developing and released, the woman can be helped with either tablets or injections. An x-ray called hysterosalpingogram (HSG) is performed to judge whether the tubes are open or not. If they are not open, they may sometimes be opened up by a radiological procedure or surgery. Alternatively, the woman may need a test tube baby procedure or IVF (in vitro fertilisation). If the uterus is not of a proper shape or size, surgery may help to normalise it. If the uterus is absent or rudimentary, the options are adoption or surrogacy.

Sometimes, the man may have the desire but is not able to perform. He may need help with medications to treat impotence or absence of ejaculation. If the sperm count is very low or the forward motility defective, medications may help. A zero sperm count may need a sperm donor or sometimes assisted reproduction. If there are sperms in the testes that are not being released into seminal fluid, they may be retrieved for fertilisation by special techniques.

Thus, infertility has a wide variety of causes and therefore multiple modes of treatment options are available.

The least invasive procedure that could be recommended based on the severity of the problem is intrauterine insemination (IUI). In intrauterine insemination, the male partner is asked to collect his semen by masturbation. This semen sample is treated in the andrology laboratory. The best sperms are loaded into a fine catheter and then injected into the woman's uterus. This is an OPD or outpatient department procedure which optimises fertility.

If the semen quality is too poor to be treated by intrauterine insemination, the couple will have to resort to in vitro fertilisation (IVF) or a test tube baby procedure. Sometimes there are a few sperms in the testes but none in the ejaculate. Such people too can be offered IVF where the sperms are extracted from the testes and then used for IVF. Depending on the factors that are detected, the couple is treated and in most cases, will have conceived after getting adequate medical guidance.

Medical science has progressed enough to largely solve the problems it can detect. Fewer people are going childless without choice. Most people may not see success in one cycle of treatment and may require another cycle, but it does usually work out. Having a child is not impossible, even though at times, it may take a lot longer than one had hoped.

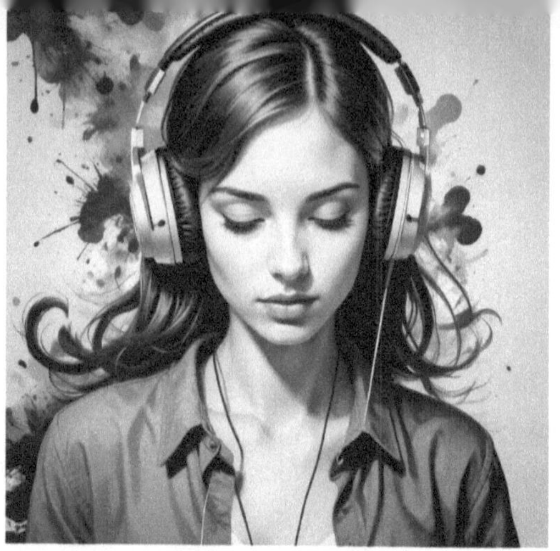

Chapter 17

DISCRETIONARY LISTENING THROUGH THE PREGNANCY

Nitya's marriage wasn't ideal. She and her husband didn't really share the same wavelength. The obvious solution her mother and mother-in-law both proposed was to have a baby as soon as possible. Since she didn't know better, she agreed. Since her husband, Subashish, didn't know better, he agreed as well. And they started trying. If nothing else, the sex was good. And they were both fertile and got lucky. So wham! They were pregnant. Now, although they usually had very little they agreed on, one thing they began to agree upon was how they should go about the pregnancy and that they would love to have a baby girl. The other thing they both soon started really feeling for together was the mountain of advice they were receiving as soon-to-be parents. She kept being told what to do and what not to do. He kept being told what to let her do and what not to let her do. Since the inception of their marriage, they weren't used to interfering in each other's day-to-day activities, and the insistence on suddenly doing everything together wasn't going to work for them. But they didn't know how to deal with it all.

There are a lot of funny things about pregnancies and babies. The ones about babies you can binge-watch on YouTube channels, but the funny stuff about pregnancy, no one has a channel for! Like, getting pregnant is really hard for someone who desperately wants to have a baby but terribly easy and accidental for someone who has no plans of getting pregnant! And one of the most ridiculous things about pregnancy is that everyone, whether or not related to you and whether or not qualified to give it to you, will give you tons of advice.

This is a tough one, isn't it? All of us are surrounded by purportedly well-meaning family, friends, acquaintances, neighbours and random strangers who start going "Oh, that's wonderful!" at the mention of an ongoing pregnancy and take it as their birthright to shower you with tons of "helpful" advice. They're pretty damn sure that because you chose to get pregnant, you must have absolutely no common sense and must need the most basic of advice administered to you repeatedly like a multivitamin. You might be smart enough to find somewhere to hide but I sure didn't! If you don't manage to run and hide, you'll really have a tough time trying to figure out how to shut them out!

Scary? I hear you. Been there, done that; or actually been told to do this and that. I mean, imagine, women who had had one kid were dishing out advice to me when I was on my third pregnancy and despite knowing fully well that I had been through the process twice before. I mean, really, what are your chances of escaping this, right?

So, learn how to deal with it. Firstly, try to ignore them. Yeah. If you have thick skin and the magical power of being able to look like you're listening while not listening at all, by all means, just pretend. It works like a charm. No harm done. Your sanity is in place, and you've managed not to offend anyone. If you are not blessed with this magical power, then try just saying "Okay, I'll try it." This works better than arguing or trying to get them to see your point. If you argue or talk back, it gives them the opportunity to drag the conversation longer and hence give you more unwanted advice. But if you just nod your head dumbly and walk off, voila! It's done! The monologue is over, and you can go back to your business.

If that doesn't help, try my trusted ABC of discretionary listening. Avoid, Bypass, Confuse. How, you ask? Let me explain.

Start avoiding the people you know are most likely to start dishing out advice the moment they lay eyes on you or your baby bump. Out of sight is out of reach, which means you stay as far away as you can from their sermons. It's a healthier approach simply because not only does it save your peace of mind, but it also prevents you from wasting your precious energy on fretting over why people can't just let you be.

For those you can't avoid, try Bypassing them. Since clearly you can't seem to control your expressions and look like you're on the verge of clawing their eyes out every time they open their mouths, try not to give in to the temptation of setting off on a rampage. Instead, say a firm no. Tell them succinctly and without going into a long tirade, that you will do as you please. This works with people who don't have a direct influence over you and your life – non-family and friends and colleagues. People basically who have no bearing on your life and just happen to be there. You can't really afford to alienate the rest.

For people who don't fall in the A and B categories, there's the blanket "C" category, meaning Confuse. Since you can't get away from them and you're in no position to retort, and clearly you have no control over your emotions, at least try to use your gift of the gab to reply funnily or indirectly in such a way that the person doesn't get the message, doesn't get hurt or offended but at least you've vented your frustration. This works really well for me with people who don't have a good knowledge of idioms and axioms. Even a simple "if you say so" serves the purpose if said on the aside without the intended audience having actually heard it. And if they ask you if you said something, you can just give a nod of your angelic head and pretend that you wouldn't dare interrupt their words of divine wisdom.

Sometimes, it's just possible someone's giving you sound advice, but the deluge of unsolicited wisdom around you will cause you to neglect the good stuff as well. Like one of the best pieces of parenting advice I received was from a friend of my cousin's co-sister! I dropped by her boutique once to buy a dress for an upcoming festival and ended up chatting with her. She was quite sympathetic about the fact that since I had just delivered my first child, I wasn't fitting into any clothes I already owned, and then proceeded to tell me a very simple thing – if you want your child to eat by themselves, serve your plate along with theirs and make sure you eat with them. That way, your child understands that eating is something that everyone must do, and they must do it themselves. Moreover, when they see that you are eating the same food you've given them, the child is more likely to adapt to that kind of food and will stop harassing you about the food you give them. I followed this sage piece of advice, and it made my life so much easier than my friends.' Every so often I think of her and thank my stars that I dropped by her shop that day!

Another thing I think I should point out is that you'd be better off not having said anything mean or wrong rather than to regret it. Whether you like it or not, you're constantly going to be anxious about how things are going for your baby and whether you're getting everything right. This will make you vulnerable to people who sound convincing although they don't know what the hell they're talking about. Similarly, it'll make you resistant to people who actually mean well and are giving you relevant insights on your pregnancy and child. So why not just listen to them and still follow your heart?

My own uncle once launched into a long discourse on how women should sweep and swab the house through their pregnancies to aid them in having a vaginal birth. I'm big to begin with, and pregnancy is hardly a good time to lose weight. This conventional piece of advice is suited to ladies who're physically fit enough to do it but not someone with weak ankles or a low-lying placenta! So yeah, be careful who you listen to.

Another trick you could try to get out of sticky situations is to come up with smart, valid excuses to cut the conversation. For example, people know you're pregnant and need frequent washroom breaks. If the conversation is becoming too much for you, the bathroom is a great place to escape to. Similarly, you are bound to be constantly hungry and thirsty. Why not just put these people on the job and send them off for a snack or a glass of water? Since they're clearly so concerned about you and your baby, they're most likely to feel obliged to run to help the mommy-to-be satiate her "pregnancy cravings."

I've come up with random things like wanting popsicles, caramel popcorn, and missal in the middle of conversations just to get people off my back. If it meant they were going to launch into another lecture on how that stuff wasn't healthy for us (the baby and me), then I've asked them to make me a sandwich and get me coconut water. Believe me, nobody says no. Not a chance. If they don't want to do it themselves, at least your request will divert their attention to them trying to get someone else to do your bidding. Not only did I end up getting pampered in the process, but it often meant that these people were wary of hanging out around me on the off-chance that I'll demand random stuff that they'll have to spend money and effort on getting me!

I also found that telling people you have a headache or that your back was aching were also effective, credible excuses for getting out of unpleasant situations through your pregnancy and for a while thereafter. Since more often than not it's also true that your head is aching and your back is killing you, it's only a smart thing to do and get some rest as often as you can while you can. I've been able to escape long religious rituals and noisy ceremonies while getting the yummy food served first through my pregnancies. Once you learn to leverage it, it becomes a fun period.

A word of caution. Don't use the privilege of pregnancy to bother your loved ones. They're already dealing with a lot, and you adding to their burden unnecessarily won't make their lives easier or make them love you more for sure. Better to reserve this for people who deserve it. That rhymes! Reserve, deserve. Get the drift?!!

So yeah. You can crib about how much everyone wants to go on and on, or you can find a way to fix it. I'm sure I've given you enough idea that you can improvise on!

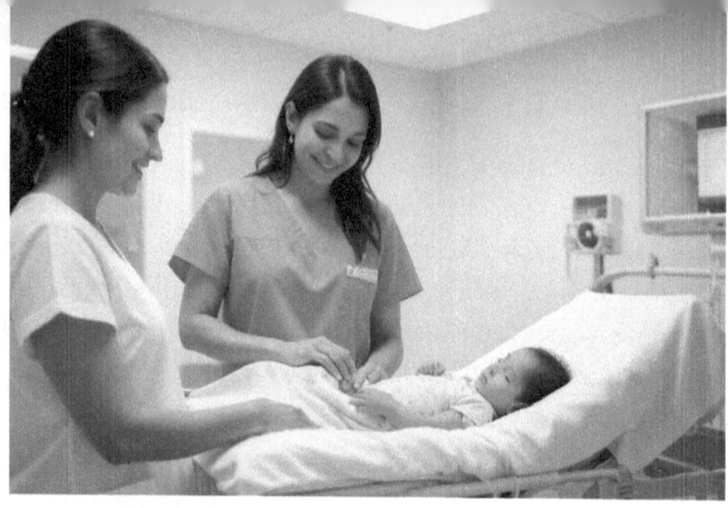

Chapter 18

DELIVERY

In 2014, when I was expecting my eldest child, I started researching the whole delivery process. I had heard of something called a water birth and thought I should figure out if it happens in India. I was told that it's not an old concept in India and though it is a good idea and widely practised abroad, I got really excited about it. It was what celebs like Gwyneth Paltrow and Gisele Bundchen had done as far back as 2005. So it must definitely be the coolest way to give birth!

Alas! Neither my dreams of a water birth nor those of a normal delivery were to be. When my baby was due and I had gone for a scan very close to my expected due date, we realised that her heartbeat had become erratic and the doctor recommended an emergency C-section to avoid any risk to the baby. All went well, and I came home with a long cut below my abdomen and a few stitches to keep it all together, and of course, a beautiful baby!

As a high school student, I loved biology, but was terribly awkward whenever I read about the reproductive anatomy of human beings. As a result, I didn't have the guts to go web-search about it for fear that my mother would wonder why! So, I grew up knowing precious little about how babies are actually ejected or removed from a woman's body! Weird? My limited research on the subject told me that most people actually share my ignorance. If you're like me, welcome to the club!

There are actually different types of delivery. You might have heard about natural birth, prolonged labour, water births, and caesarean sections, but might not really know what each means and what they are really about. Let me tell you a little about them now.

As you're aware, the baby lies in the mother's uterus for a period of 9 months to grow from a speck of dirt into an actual being with hands and legs and a nose and 2 eyes and 2 ears. Delivery is the process by which the baby comes out of the mother's body. This can happen in 2 ways really and either way, the process takes a huge toll on the mother's body. The unfortunate thing is, after the delivery, the care a mother receives is far lesser than what she received through the pregnancy.

Firstly, what is labour? Labour is the physiological process by which the baby and all that stuff it was swimming in, in the mother's uterus come out of the mother's body. Labour is painful because it requires the cervix of the mother's body to expand enough to allow a full baby to come out of it. The cervix is the lower part of the uterus which connects to the vagina. Normally, a cervix is only about an inch long and rigid, and it is closed. During pregnancy, the cervix softens and shortens in order to aid the passage of the baby. Imagine something as big as a -2.5kilogram watermelon passing through it. The kind of pain that entails is what a mother goes through during labour and vaginal birth.

When you go for your pre-natal classes, you'll hear a lot about vaginal birth, why you should exercise, do a lot of squats, practice kegel exercises, etc. I think you should know that there is no best-known way to have a baby. No one way is the one best way. "Natural birth" is an unfair term. The birth of a baby is a natural phenomenon. At the same time, there's nothing "natural" left in the birth of babies any more. I mean, what's natural about taking medicines for a healthy mother or a healthy baby or for getting pregnant or taking injections to avoid a disease or anything associated with medicine? So why talk about something happening the way God meant it to happen and all that when really nothing is working the way it was meant to work!

What people mean when they speak about 'natural birth' is a vaginal birth. A vaginal birth is the process of the baby coming out of the mother's vagina once it's ready to come out and the mother is in labour. The duration of your labour depends on how much your cervix has dilated, i.e., expanded, to allow the baby to come out, and how quickly that happens. The duration of labour is subjective and contrary to whatever people tell you, largely out of your control. No matter how much you exercise and consume ghee in milk, there's no guarantee you'll pop your baby out in a few minutes!

I have tons of stories of labour. My own sister-in-law went through 22 hours of labour before she finally couldn't try to push anymore, and the doctor took a call that they should do a C-section to avoid any complications. The ordeal left her traumatised for a while, and she deferred her second pregnancy just so that she didn't have to go through it again, and even at that, she decided to opt for a planned surgery to avoid the stress.

A lady I learnt yoga from for a few months has another interesting story. A lot of people believe that consuming castor oil once your contractions have begun helps to push the baby out quickly. In her case, the castor oil caused the baby to poop in the womb, and as soon as the doctor realised something was off, she was operated on to deliver the baby. Not only did all her plans for a normal delivery go out of the window, but there were some minor complications eventually as well. While it does happen even if you don't consume castor oil, the ingestion of these stools is not necessarily fatal for the baby. Having said that, you don't want to do anything to jeopardise the health of your child, and you cannot control whether you will have a so-called natural delivery or not.

A caesarean section means removing the baby from the mother's uterus by cutting open her lower abdomen. It is done under local anaesthesia and takes about half an hour. Your gynaecologist will brief you and your partner and make you sign a few forms before they complete the process and eventually hand you the baby from across the screen that is used to cover the lower half of your body. Again, like with vaginal deliveries, each lady's body performs differently during the C-section, and your experience might not be the same as someone else.

I was lucid through all 3 of my C-sections and had a chat with my surgeon on the deteriorated state of my uterus during the last one before she finally showed me my son! One of the worst horror stories about a C-section is that of my husband's cousin's wife. She was undergoing a C-section for her second child, who was too big to be pushed out. The doctor administered the anaesthesia, but something clearly didn't work because she felt the knife cut through the 7 layers of tissue that the scalpel went through! It's the only such case I'm aware of, and I've heard a truckload of stories, but it's something that gives me goosebumps even today!

You'll hear from people how great it is to have a "natural delivery," and they'll go on and on about it forever. I've been in labour once for 6 hours and swore off it then and there. My next 2 were scheduled C-sections, and dare anyone tell me that I'm any less of a mother for not having pushed my babies out of my vagina! The first time, I did try, but my baby got her leg entangled in the umbilical cord, and her heartbeat kept fluctuating on the foetal heartbeat monitor. So my doctor took a call and pulled her out to avoid taking a risk. And it was done.

If you have the endurance and your doctor suggests it, try your best for a vaginal birth. It will mean fewer stitches than what you get during a C-section. After a vaginal birth, usually, the doctor will have to stitch your cervix back together. The stitches will take a while to heal, and you'll have a bit of difficulty sitting properly on your backside, but that's fine. Eventually, it'll all be alright. Your doctor will have to take into consideration your risk profile while deciding whether or not you can try for a vaginal birth. Your risk profile will include your age, weight, any prior history of miscarriage, etc. Also, a vaginal birth is not considered a full-blown surgery and is cheaper. But get whatever medical advice you must because it may or may not be for you.

If you have to have a caesarean section, it will mean a quick surgery cutting through 7 layers of tissue in the abdomen to finally reach that little baby you've waited so long for. Not enough people understand that a C-section is a complex surgery and while it is really common these days, it is still a surgery and a major one at that. Once the surgeon has removed your baby and drained out all that is no longer required inside your uterus, he/she will stitch your uterus back together and put a dressing that'll allow you to function fairly normally once you've recovered. There will be a lot of pain for a while but they'll give you medication to deal with it. Again, you'll be fine, eventually.

There is an increasing noise about water birthing. Water birthing means going through labour while sitting in a pool or tub of water. It is considered less painful. I did some research about it, but eventually, our family wasn't sure it was a good idea, and I had to ditch it. Not that I was going to have a vaginal delivery anyway!

Don't get into debates on which one is better. No one type is the best for everyone. Something that works for you may not work for someone else. Some people don't have the option to make a choice. Someone may have scheduled a C-section and gone into labour prematurely. Someone who tried their best to have a vaginal birth may have a complication leading to a surgical birth. It doesn't matter so long as both the mother and child are fine, right? It's easier to preach when you're on a side of the fence far away from the border. I believe one shouldn't preach even if you went through one or the other. You don't know someone else's battles.

I was visiting my gynaecologist for a post-op visit after my second daughter when I saw this really beautiful lady sitting on the sofa opposite me in the waiting room at the hospital. She looked really fit, although it was obvious her baby wasn't more than a few weeks old. I was inwardly cursing my genes for making me a soft, plump slob who would need to spend thousands of hours in the gym and maybe truckloads of money to look like her. A few minutes later, she changed her seat and sat beside me, and we got talking. I found out that she, this beautiful goddess who seemed so perfect, was a type-I diabetic who had been taking insulin injections since the age of 14. Throughout her pregnancy, she had to take double the dose of her regular insulin just so that the baby would survive. It had been an unexpected pregnancy, a really difficult one, and her doctor (the same as mine) had told her clearly there should never be another! I really learnt that no one has it all and nobody's life is perfect that day. I felt a little ashamed of my own feelings. Eventually, I realised that the only way to be happy is to be grateful for what you have.

Having a baby is a beautiful thing and it is such a privilege. Dissecting this privilege is a pathetic thing to do. Don't let people who comment on how you should go about having your child get to you. Let your body be your guide and let the experts help you determine what might or might not be correct for you.

As a co-parent, you must be aware of all this and also the fact that the mother is going to need as much care and attention as the newborn. She's just been through tons of pain and is probably going to be in pain for a while to come. Her body's just changed so much that she'll probably never recognise herself as her old self again. She's coming to terms with consciously feeding an individual from her body, at whose beck and call she must be. She's careworn, sleep-deprived, and clueless. Be gentle. Be considerate. Be there for her. That you are both now parents is enough. Celebrate and give as much as you can to each other because it happened. Eventually, how it happened will only be a footnote in your history as a parent.

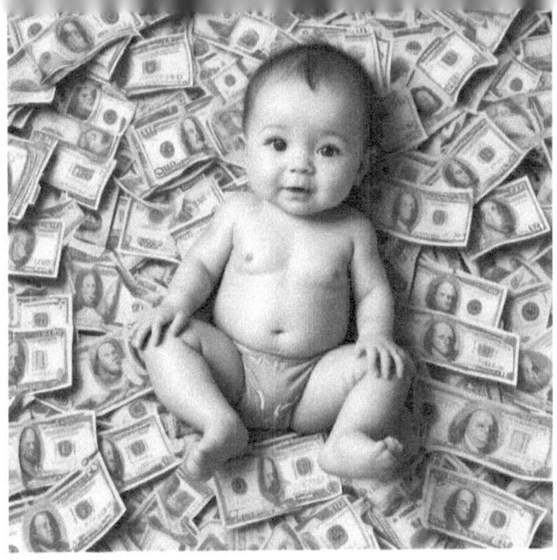

Chapter 19

WHAT IT COSTS TO RAISE A CHILD

Lekha and Sujeet run a restaurant. It is a small, cosy place in a nice part of Mumbai. They're diligent, friendly, and the food at their restaurant is really excellent. They had a small part of their office converted into a nursery for their daughter. So they were able to care for her through her pre-school life without too much trouble because at least one of them would be at the restaurant all day. By the time Covid-19 struck, their daughter, Anaisha, was in grade 1 and would come directly to the restaurant after school. But soon, they had to shut shop because of the pandemic. While they had a good business going, the premises were on rent and with zero sales, there was no chance of sustaining the cost of keeping the business going. On the other hand, their personal finances also weren't great because they hadn't really thought ahead enough to make hay while the sun shone. That year, paying Anaisha's hefty school fee was also a challenge.

They fired all their help and cut back on non-essential expenses to make it through the difficult period. Luckily, their landlord let them take the place back on after the restrictions were relaxed and though gradually they built their business back brick-by-brick, they had learnt a lot of lessons the hard way.

Most people don't seriously start thinking about how expensive life in general is these days because their parents foot their cost of living. It's only when they move out and start living on their own that reality sets in. Even then, if you are fending for yourself alone and have no other obligations, things can be a lot of fun. Spending on expensive gadgets, branded clothes and extravagant holidays is part of the course.

For those who buy a home using a loan, things do tend to change. You might not have even tried any kind of discipline in finance until you had those EMIs coming in every month. The mortgage on a bike or car is far lesser in money terms than that on a house. So where your monthly instalments on the vehicle didn't make a major dent in your finances perhaps, the instalments of your home loan are definitely bound to affect your lifestyle. Therefore, if you've gotten used to planning your finances around your unavoidable cash outflow, you are going to find it a little easier to alter your budget to accommodate your child.

The expenses don't wait for your child to be born. Like I mentioned in chapter 10, the meter starts from the moment you get serious about having the baby. This is only part of the game. Raising a child in India is pretty expensive these days, and as per various studies that I have used for reference, the cost of raising a child from childhood up to post-graduation is approximately Rs. 60 lakhs in 2020. The figure keeps increasing depending on the rate of inflation. If you choose to provide more expensive education, then you need to tailor your numbers to reflect that. This is an average cost in a tier1-city.

In the first 2 years of a child alone, you need to spend a big chunk of money on paediatrician visits and vaccinations. This can end up being as much as Rs. 75,000 for a child from birth up to 2 years. The visits to the doctor are pretty frequent during the first 2 years of a child's life even for a completely healthy child, but children tend to have low immunity in their first few years, and since typically first-time parents are not sure of how to deal with even minor ailments like coughs and colds, they tend to rush to the doctor for everything.

Another cost that a lot of working parents have no choice but to incur these days is that of a day care or nanny. If you want a full-day help, it will cost you a minimum of Rs. 10,000 per month in most tier 1 and 2 cities. All of these things, though critical for your convenience and comfort, do make a draw on your pockets. So being aware is important. Even if you don't have someone to monitor the child and opt for day care services, you will still be forking out about the same amount of money.

The approximate cost of raising a child up to 2 years of age is detailed in the table below:

Particulars	Frequency	Cost/unit	Amt (Rs.)
Paediatrician visits (assuming once in 3 months other than vaccination)	8	500	4,000
Mandatory vaccines	12	2,500	30,000
Other medicines and nutritional supplements	24	1,500	36,000
Diapers	24	500	12,000
Toys			25,000
Massage person	12	2,000	24,000
Nanny	24	10,000	240,000

Particulars	Frequency	Cost/unit	Amt (Rs.)
Birthday Parties for the child	2	10,000	20,000
Gifts for other kids' birthday parties	6	500	3,000
Apparel			30,000
Accessories for the Baby (Stroller, walker, baby chair, bedding)			32,000
Total			456,000

After 2 years of age, the cost of vaccinations and massage personnel will be replaced by a number of other costs. Since the parents may be working full-time, they may opt for day care services, which at a bare minimum work out to Rs. 12,000 per month. The cost of vaccinations comes down, but as the child's exposure to the outside world increases, the child tends to fall sick more often as his immunity is not that strong. Overall, the cost of raising the child up to 5 years of age, i.e., getting the child through pre-primary school, would look like this:

Particulars	Per annum	Total (Rs.) for 3 years
Reputed private preschool fees	50,000	150,000
Vaccination and treatment for routine illnesses	20,000	60,000
Apparel	20,000	60,000
Nutritional supplements	24,000	72,000
Toys, books and stationery	10,000	30,000
Nanny/daycare	144,000	432,000
Birthday Parties/Playzone visits/ Other events	25,000	75,000
Total		879,000

Eventually, the tapering cost of vaccinations and doctor visits will be replaced by the increasing cost of education and extracurricular learning. Since the focus on building fine arts skills and advanced abilities in STEM (Science, Technology, Engineering, and Maths) is so high, the incidence of extra classes is also higher than it used to be. So, while the basket of spending may change, the overall annual cost of raising the child doesn't decline. The total cost of raising a single child from 8-3 years of age would look like this:

Particulars	Per annum	Total (Rs.) for 3 years
Education	60,000	180,000
Extra-curricular and co-curricular classes	24,000	72,000
Vaccinations and routine doctor's visits	12,000	36,000
Nutritional supplements & food	40,000	120,000
Apparel & accessories	30,000	90,000
Toys, books and stationery	30,000	90,000
Nanny/daycare	144,000	432,000
Birthday Parties/Playzone visits/ Other events	25,000	75,000
Total		1,095,000

The total annual expenditure will largely remain on an upward trajectory throughout a child's life. The way things are these days, it is near-impossible to not incur a lot of expense on extra and co-curricular classes. As the child gets older and their immunity improves, the cost of doctor's visits and vaccinations reduces, but the cost of books and stationery increases. Further, as the child becomes old enough to not need a caretaker/nanny, that cost is reduced, but children this age typically need to be given some money to spend when they are away from the parents, and this becomes their pocket money. Since the children spend most of their time during this period in uniforms, the cost of clothing and accessories doesn't increase significantly. The major addition is the increase in the cost of extra classes, be it tuitions or extracurricular classes.

Particulars	Per annum	Total (Rs.) for 4 years
Education	60,000	240,000
Extra-curricular classes and tuitions	48,000	192,000
Vaccinations and routine doctor's visits	6,000	24,000
Nutritional supplements & food	30,000	120,000
Apparel & accessories	30,000	120,000
Books and stationery	40,000	160,000
Pocket Money	6,000	24,000
Birthday Parties/Playzone visits/Other events	50,000	200,000
Total		1,080,000

The costs from the pre-teen period to the completion of high school remain reasonably stable except the cost of tuitions and the child's added expenditure on matching their peer group's lifestyle. While this is hard to calculate, I have taken a rough benchmark to give you an idea of what the numbers will look like. Tuitions in the last couple of years of school are very expensive these days as the pressure to perform well in board exams and entrance tests is very high. Further, as children grow older, their needs change and the money they need is also more. You have to factor all of this into your planning. The cost of raising the child through teenage upto 18 years will look like this:

Particulars	Per annum	Total (Rs.) for 6 years
Education	70,000	420,000
Extra-curricular and co-curricular classes	60,000	360,000
Vaccinations and routine doctor's visits	6,000	36,000
Nutritional supplements & food	30,000	180,000
Apparel & accessories	40,000	240,000
Toys, books and stationery	60,000	360,000
Pocket Money	9,600	57,600
Birthday Parties/Playzone visits/ Other events	50,000	300,000
Total		1,953,600

Add up all the tables, and the total is quite significant. At my estimates for someone who is probably considered middle to upper-middle class in India, the cost of raising a child up to 18 years of age is around Rs. 54.63 lakhs. This is only a suggestive figure based on estimates for tier-II cities in India. It is enough to help you set the right expectations in terms of what you will need to be earning to be able to raise your child comfortably.

I can never stress enough the importance of being organised in your approach to medical care. People often feel that we'll cross the bridge when we come to it, but what they don't realise until it's too late is that not only would they have saved an extraordinary amount of money by planning ahead and ensuring they prepared in advance for unforeseen medical expenses, but also that they would save themselves a great deal of stress and headache. This is even more relevant to those who live alone and in big cities with little or no help.

We live in times of uncertainty, and you never know what can happen. While we live like we're going to be on the earth forever, it is really important that we plan for the future bearing in mind that we do have a finite shelf life. Invest from an early age and plan your expenses keeping in mind that your needs are never going to be fewer. In youth, your medical needs are fewer but desire for life is great. In old age, it is the opposite; so what you spent earlier on having a good life you will eventually spend on making sure your life is not difficult. Either way, it will be important to be self-sufficient and not dependent on anyone.

The same applies to your responsibilities towards your children. What the insurance companies get right is this – that life is uncertain and that we must plan for every eventuality. Learn about policies that will help cover your various risks and obligations and build the financial discipline that it takes to keep all these things in good shape. Discipline in your personal and financial health will both aid in keeping you on top of things, as a parent and as an individual. When you choose to have a child, do it responsibly and knowing fully well exactly what you are getting into. The choice at the end of the day is yours. And you want it to be something that'll add happiness to your life. So, it's worthwhile to ensure that you work towards it with the right mindset and expectations, whether emotionally, physically or financially.

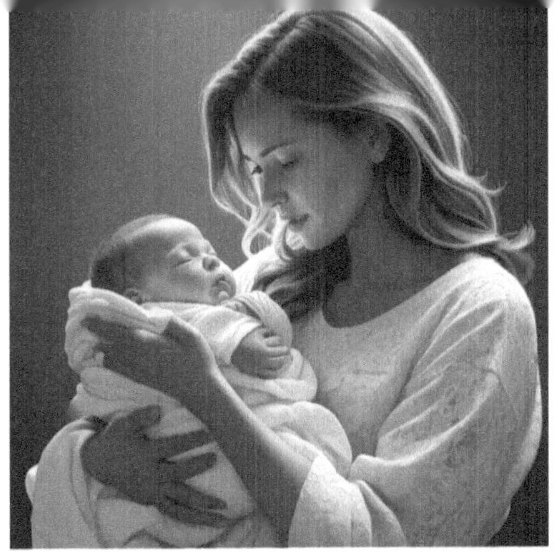

Chapter 20

DEALING WITH THE NEWBORN AND THE NEW MOM

Sunny is true to his name. His disposition is bright, and he tends to be the one bringing any party to life. He was used to a reasonably carefree life throughout, but that didn't mean he was careless. He took his wedding vows seriously and made sure to live up to the expectation of his lady love. His relationship with his wife, Neha, was solid because of the commonalities between them. But this didn't last forever. The birth of their son, Krish, changed Neha rather suddenly and drastically. Always one to be game for an outing or adventure, suddenly Neha became irritable and bitter. She wasn't the person Sunny had married, and although in his mind he was doing everything it took to ensure that she and the baby were comfortable, he had no idea that in her mind, she was fighting a lone battle in figuring out life after childbirth. There was a full-time jaapa maid and all the latest gadgets were there – the breast pump, feeding pillow, baby bouncer and soothing musical toys. But what weren't there according to Neha were her own familiar body, the ability to do things at will and the rest of a night's undisturbed sleep. Sunny failed to understand any of this because he simply didn't know better, and Neha's limited fault was that she didn't make the effort to explain any of it to him.

The pain and longing that you've been through for 9 months at the very, very least will finally come to an end the moment you meet a very special person for the first time – your baby. That moment will be etched in your minds forever. It is something that you worked hard for and felt like you had waited on for just so long. But that will not be all.

You will feel great trepidation and fear about how you are dealing with this special being. Every moment will be a first. There will be many mistakes to make and much to learn! So how do you go about all of it without feeling underwhelmed by how unprepared you truly are after all that effort you put in? Nothing would have prepared you for the first few days of parenthood in entirety, for the actual experience.

First off, let me tell you, all those classes and books you read were not for nothing. Not at all. But see, there's a difference between reading a driving instruction booklet and finally actually driving a car. The same goes for parenting. The knowledge is helpful and relevant and gives you some idea of what's actually up with your baby. At the same time, because you went for those classes and learnt those things, while you may not be prepared for everything, you know more than before. So don't dish those experiences.

Even if you don't read any books on it and don't do any classes, a lot of it will come to you naturally. We have an inner nurturer and a natural instinct for being protectors and caretakers. These instincts guide us and help us become parents without the real need for too much help. However, there are complicated things that we are likely to know about only if informed. So learn to use the 2 things in tandem - external instruction and your natural parenting instincts. Learn to rely on each as and when the need arises and figure out the correct balance.

Your fears are only natural. You've never been a parent before. You may not have held a baby in your arms even, let alone be responsible for it. Even if you've held someone else's child, the delicate connection with your own flesh and blood is a different thing altogether. It throws your senses out of gear and makes you so vulnerable. Every inch of your being feels each cry of your baby like a dagger through your soul, and every hiccup is like a tsunami warning. Calm down. It's not. The worst that can happen is you'll spend a sleepless night and end up harrowing your paediatrician so many times that she'll start charging you by the minute.

When I was expecting my eldest baby, I thought I would be the calmest mother ever. The coolest one. Fast forward to day 2 of being a mom, in the wee hours of the morning, after breastfeeding my darling daughter non-stop for almost 2 hours, I couldn't seem to get her to sleep or get any sleep myself. Sleep-deprived and with my senses dulled by pain medication, I turned into a momster. I called for the head nurse on duty and asked her why the hell my baby refused to sleep. Wasn't I feeding her enough or had the nurse who'd changed the baby's diapers not put them on properly? I complained that maybe the quantity of food they'd given me that day wasn't enough and maybe that was why my baby hadn't gotten enough milk and that's why she was unable to sleep! I went on and on for almost an hour. They had to call the nursing department head. She just told me to hang in there until my doctor came in.

Eventually when my gynaecologist came in, I got a simple talk down from her. While she didn't exactly admonish me for losing it so unceremoniously at someone who was only trying to help me, she did have a hearty laugh at my expense and told me that a few years down the line, I would be laughing at my old self too. I learnt that day that I was never going to be a cool and calm mom. I was destined to be the worst kind that would worry at every sneeze and flip at every cough. I was going to be one of those "weird moms" I once showered my precious condescension on. I was the worst sugar syrupy kind of mom I never wanted to be!

Eventually, I did learn to stop running to the paediatrician for every minor thing. With my second child, the number of visits to the doctor came down by almost half, and by the third, to a quarter. It took time, and I learnt that children do fall, they do cry, they do have sleepless nights. So do you. You will have days when you'll question your parenting skills and days when you'll wonder how wise it was to have had a kid at all. You'll think that it will never get better through the first few days of your first child. You'll be in pain and will deal with the anguish that comes because your child is unwell or you didn't meet the growth chart targets and you'll beat yourself blue for every petty thing. Eventually, someday, you will laugh at the new mom that you were. Dealing with a newborn needs calm hands as well. Let those around you take over if you can't seem to hold yourself together. Handle the baby alone and let everyone else do their job. There are people to handle your nutrition, people to ensure that your baby is properly bathed and changed and inoculated. You'll cringe at the thought of someone sticking in a needle in your precious little's arm, but rest assured it's for her good. Don't shy away from asking questions. Everyone understands. They may not necessarily be patient, but they owe it to you to answer your questions.

So ask away.

I've had some really funny incidents in my time as a parent.

I was taking my eldest for the first time to Bangalore, where my parents live. I had bought a baby sling so that I could handle her more comfortably in the flight and since she was already 3 months old, I was told it was safe to put her into it. At the check-in counter, a woman who looked to be around a few years older than me, kept giving me these funny looks. My daughter was crying and since I was carrying her in the baby sling, I kept swaying her from side to side to help soothe her. I couldn't imagine what was so funny about me doing that, that the lady couldn't stop looking at us. Finally, after 20 minutes, the lady walked up to us and without a word, adjusted the harness at the back. Apparently, I was carrying my kid way too long because of which she just staring at my torso. I hadn't known how much to shorten the harness, resulting in this gaffe.

As soon as she was at my neck level, she stopped crying because she could now see my face! I felt really foolish at that point but was really grateful for the help.

Even after I got to Bangalore, I got into a fix. I had been there about a week. My daughter had pooped the day we arrived and it had been 4 days since and no potty! I knew that up to 6 months, this is pretty common when the child is exclusively breastfed. I was beginning to panic and finally called our paediatrician. She asked me to get something called a suppository. It's a glycerin capsule that helps the baby poop and you're supposed to insert it into the rectum in order to do that. I misunderstood what the doctor said and was about to give it to my daughter orally when my mom stopped me. She said the kid would gag on such a big capsule and that I must've gotten it wrong. Thankfully, I called the doc again and asked her what to do with it. Can you imagine what could've happened had I tried to feed the medicine to the child?!!!

Another facility available these days is a lactation expert. Who's that, you want to know? A lactation expert is someone who knows how to breastfeed the baby. She will teach you everything from how to hold the child and what position is best for you to what you should eat to ensure a healthy breast milk supply. A lactation expert has become relevant in our times because we simply don't live in families. Earlier, your older cousin or your brother's wife would help you out because your mother would've been out of the breastfeeding business for way too long. Since most people either don't have someone to help out or aren't comfortable asking family, a lactation expert is a good option. You can also have them come home after discharge if you're still having a hard time getting your baby to latch onto you and feed properly.

A few questions that most families grapple with and that become a bone of contention between modern medicine and traditional beliefs deserve mention here. The first one will be whether you can have some outsider massage your baby and if yes, what oil should be used. While almost all doctors will tell you that unless you yourself are planning on massaging your baby, there's no need to get a professional masseuse for your child, your mother or mother-in-law will insist you get one. These ladies are also good at giving the baby a bath, will swaddle the child, help you give the baby any medication prescribed by the doctor and rock the baby to sleep once all of that is done. I got one for each of my kids and don't regret the decision. The choice, however, is yours.

The other common question is what oil to use. It really depends on the time of the year your child was born. Some oils have a heating tendency, and some are considered cold oils. This means that some oils, if used in summer, could cause the delicate skin of your baby to break out in boils. A cold oil is considered to be better in the summer. That would, for example, include coconut oil. Mustard oil is considered a hot oil and is often used in monsoons and winters as it also helps when the child has a cold or cough. I've used a combination of oils depending on the season and my baby's skin. You won't have answers to all of these questions on day 1 but there's plenty of help out there. Even a lot of social media mother support groups tend to give us the kind of information books generally don't have.

Let your baby be your guide in a lot of decisions. Children can actually tell us silently in their own way what they want or don't. If your baby is crying, it's usually only for 1 out of 5 reasons – she's hungry, she's sleepy, she's colicky, she's pooped or she just wants to be held. First, check her diaper. If she's not pooped or her diaper's not full, try feeding, putting her to sleep or carrying her around for a bit. If none of these works, try giving your baby a small dose of whatever colic medication your paediatrician's prescribed and you should be fine. It's trial and error. There's no magic indicator on the kid that tells you what exactly is wrong. You'll figure out the patterns over a period of time. Till then, stick to trial and error. You'll realise that sometimes, the child wanted nothing more than the warmth of your arms and your time.

Don't worry. You'll get better at it. In due course of time. Soon, it'll all start coming to you naturally. When I had my eldest, people would tell me to try putting the baby to sleep or something else. I would wonder how exactly they knew what was wrong with my baby. Slowly I understood it all comes from experience. There was nothing wrong with me. I was just a first-time mother. I wasn't expected to know. No one will expect you to magically transform into the mom-of-the-decade overnight. That's why people give you advice. Sometimes, try listening to it and don't dish it right away.

You'll figure out your little human, one step at a time. Be gentle. Not only with the baby, but with yourself and your spouse. It's really hard on both of you too. There's no university that gives out PhDs on parenting. Even if they did, we'd all fail at the real-life tests because becoming a parent changes your DNA and brings to life your greatest vulnerabilities. So remind each other that it's okay and that you are doing a fine job. Remind each other that this is what you both created together. It'll all work out.

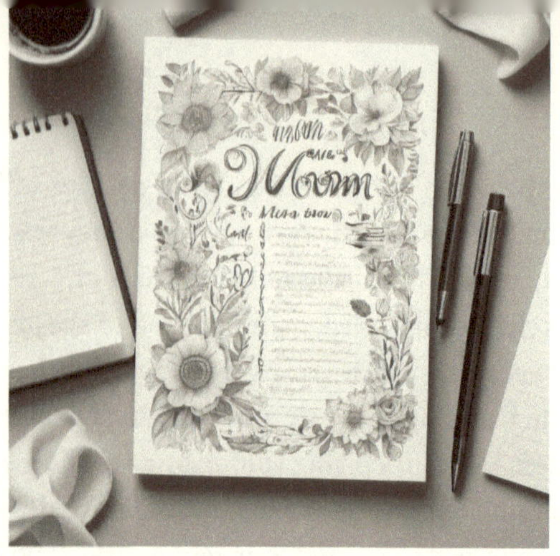

Chapter 21

IMPORTANT NOTES FOR THE FIRST FEW DAYS AFTER CHILD BIRTH

As babies go, and I'm sure all of them are cute, but one of the most beautiful and photogenic ones I've ever met is Ritwik. He looks like the cherubs made out of marble were possibly a bad imitation of him; so you can imagine! But while that was for the rest of the world, for his poor parents, he was a different matter altogether. He was born at a healthy 3.24 kilograms and came out of the tummy pretty quick. Just like his haste to come into the world, he seemed to be in a hurry to do everything the first few days. He went through his first full pack of a dozen diapers (small size mind you, not newborn) in the first 2 days of coming home. Yup, 24 diapers in 2 days. He would squirt small amounts of the terrible blackish-green poop that newborns are famous for every half an hour so and in such mysteriously weird amounts that one could neither keep him in that diaper till he pooped some more nor feel ecologically responsible for discarding it immediately. Oh, by the way, he slept through the day like an angel. The pooping seemingly happened between 11 pm and 5 am every day, till pretty much 15 days of his life.

Ritwik isn't an exception. Newborns don't come with a preset manual and they definitely don't honour any kind of code or timetable. Their freshly-baked parents lose their elation at the birth of their child at the same speed as an iPhone loses its market value the moment you unbox it! So when I say that the first few days are the toughest, believe me. The good news is that it does get better. The bad news is that not really soon though!

The first 15-10 days are the hardest, not just because you're new to the whole shebang of parenting, but also because babies don't necessarily have a timetable. A newborn may poop 10 times a day or once in 5 days. The amount of sleep I've lost, I mean practically not just rhetorically, over my kid's poop is not funny. Similarly, although newborns are supposed to sleep almost 18 hours a day, you can't predict how long their naps will be, how frequently they'll want to be fed or how often they'll wake up!

Both my older children had this horrible habit of pooping in the middle of the night, like 1:30-1 am... unearthly hours. It meant not only waking up in the middle of the night to clean them up and change their diapers but also that the whole house would wake up because they were bawling through the clean-up. Not a happy time at all. It's only after they stopped pooping at those crazy hours, did I manage to start getting some sleep in the night. I became a pro at feeding them half asleep and would sometimes not even realise how long I had fed them at night. If your kids are kind enough to not do this to you, be grateful and send a prayer up to whoever may be listening.

The colour of your baby's poop matters. Oh yeah, it's a thing. The change in the colour of a newborn's poop from almost black to green to yellow is a process and is actually a result of the removal of accumulated mucus, skin cells, and amniotic fluid from the baby's body. It's called meconium. As the body waste is flushed out, the poop gradually turns green and eventually a normal-looking yellow. The consistency of a newborn's poop is somewhat runny because newborns are on a liquid diet. So don't lose it when you see the black poop and eventually the runny yellow stuff. It's normal.

Another big query is how long should your baby feed so that her tummy is full. You can't predict. It depends on how quick a feeder your baby is and also how frequently she demands a feed. A baby who is a quick feeder and demands feeds at shorter intervals may not go over 10-5 minutes. Another may take 30 minutes to finish a meal. It's just the luck of the draw for you, which type of baby you're going to have!

Another big question mark for most mothers is with respect to using formula milk. Firstly, what is formula milk? Formula milk is a powder made from cow's milk usually and fortified to replicate to some extent human breast milk. Since it's made from cow's milk, it's not really similar to human milk but it's a substitute food, just like the milk people consume. Just like human milk is meant to meet a human child's need, cow milk is really meant to meet a calf's milk. The advances in manufacturing techniques and science aid it to provide as much nutrition as possible from an external source. While mom's milk is best, you may need to resort to formula at some point, if at all.

It's not a crime to formula-feed your child. If you aren't lactating enough, then you have no choice but to supplement your baby's diet with formula. If you're a working mother and must be away from your child for hours at a time, then you also have the option of using a breast pump to express your milk and store it for usage while you're away. The formula can act as a backup in case your milk runs out.

While the mother's milk is definitely very important for a baby, if your child isn't exclusively breastfed, you're not the worst mother on earth. Definitely try to stick to the natural as far as you can, but if it isn't enough or circumstances demand a substitute, by all means use one. No one has the right to judge you for it.

The debate over breastfeeding and how you get classified as a mother is ever-heated and raging. I know a lot of women who have resorted to formula for a variety of reasons. Some couldn't bear to stay up through the night to keep feeding repeatedly, as they had to manage either their jobs or household chores through the day. Some didn't lactate enough to be able to exclusively breastfeed. Some just couldn't bear the physical burden any longer.

A word that a lot of mothers really look forward to once they're tired of breastfeeding is weaning. Weaning is the process of getting your child onto a normal diet and off the breast. It happens gradually and needs to be worked on. Don't expect it to happen suddenly and don't try anything drastic. Caution and patience will pay off. Breastfeeding improves your child's immunity and gives you precious time to bond with your child. Someday, when your kid no longer wants to spend hours around you, you will miss these days. Make no mistake, breastfeeding is a demanding and taxing job, but it's worth it. Figure out what works for you and don't let someone's judgement bother you. It's your kid and your body. I've breastfed each of my babies for close to a year. My eldest stopped at around 13 months, while my youngest gave it up at 11 months. Not my decision at all.

I've used formula after my kids turned 3 months or more when I didn't have time to express or I was too tired to do it. I didn't let it become a substitute for my milk and made sure I took adequate calcium and iron supplements while breastfeeding to ensure my health didn't suffer and also that the baby was getting an adequate dosage of both essentials. But I only did what made me comfortable.

There were times when I would feel guilty for giving the baby one portion of formula so that I could go out for a few hours. My husband would calm me down and tell me that it's alright. He would remind me that I'm human too and that so long as I'm not ignoring my baby's needs, my actions would count as moderation. You'll feel these pangs too if you choose my route. But hey, it's your choice completely.

Pro-tip: sleep when your baby sleeps. Through the first few weeks especially when the baby doesn't have a fixed sleeping pattern, your body is going to be in really bad shape. So ditch everything else and make sure you sleep. Remember that part of the book where I told you to get a support system in place, paid or otherwise? This is what it was for. You've been through a lot physically and your life has undergone a huge transformation. You're sleep-deprived and fairly clueless about what you're doing right and what you're doing wrong. But make no mistake, you need tons of rest. Every time your baby falls asleep, don't go rushing to your phone or the gym. Sleep. Everything else can wait, and you'll have enough opportunity for catching up with the world later.

Don't start eating for 2. Just like that doesn't work in pregnancy, it doesn't pay post-partum. You need around 500 extra calories if your child is exclusively breastfed, but that's about it. Make sure you get lots of vitamins and protein in those extra calories. Don't fear to binge a little as well. For most women, breastfeeding leads to a lot of weight loss. So it may be a good time to indulge your sweet tooth or savoury cravings. That's not the case with me. I NEVER EVER lost weight because I was breastfeeding. While that doesn't mean I didn't eat what I felt like, but definitely in moderation and bearing in mind portion control. Sigh!!!

Even if you choose not to get your baby a masseuse, get yourself one. I personally recommend it. Make sure they avoid getting around your stitches and stuff, and start only after consulting your gynaec. It really helps get rid of all the pain. Your nerves have been stretched, your back is bust, your feet have carried tons of extra water, and your eyes are bloodshot. The massage will help soothe the pain and relax a really tired body and frustrated mind. Take that hour off daily as soon as possible so that you can survive. I really miss those days when I could get a massage and not feel like I was committing a crime. I felt much better after getting massaged for 15 days. Also, it helps avoid engorgement of breasts in the initial days after delivery when your baby doesn't feed a lot.

If someone offers to watch the baby or bring you a meal, let them. Express a little and go off to sleep or get the massage done. It's not selfish. To the contrary, it'll help you focus and be better at the task at hand. If someone who's in the position to help out isn't offering help, ask for it. It's alright. Better to ask than to regret not having done it. Even if they mind, they're unlikely to deny or begrudge you asking.

One of my old neighbours had her second child around the same time as I had my eldest. Her mother-in-law didn't allow her to hire a masseuse for her this time. My friend was lactating a lot from day 1 and her baby's milk needs weren't that high, as is expected from a newborn baby. She had severely engorged breasts within a week of discharge from the hospital and she was dripping milk all the time. It became so bad that when she did try to feed, she was bleeding and the milk was actually completely unpalatable. It took almost 3 weeks of regular massage, using a silicon shield and a breast pump intermittently to bring the situation under control. It was a terrible few weeks for her.

While the above situation was different, I know of cases where the mother had a tough time dealing with the changes in her own body. One of my sisters is a case in point. She was always a chubby kid and became obsessed with weight loss after she went to college. This obsession never went away. After she had her first child and was put on a jaapa diet full of ghee by her husband's grandmother, she ended up putting on 20 kgs. She went practically nuts. As soon as she finished her jaapa, she went on a strict diet and started working out. She would work out for 2.5 hours a day at a stretch, and to be able to accommodate that time, she would feed her baby a bottle full of formula milk before hitting the gym. After she returned, she'd be really exhausted and would administer another bottle of formula so that she could sleep through the night. She did lose a lot of weight and quickly. But eventually, as her son grew up, he had poor immunity. Scientifically you can't really blame the poor immunity on the bottle feeding. But she blames herself for it to date.

I know my own aunt (her mother) put this thought into her head. But I feel the blame game is unfair and useless. A lot of exclusively breastfed children also fall sick frequently. It's not just one thing. Moreover, isn't the mother's state of mind as important as the child's health? If the mother is suffering physically and mentally and needs to do something about it, you can't make her sound selfish or blame her for being a careless mother. It's a choice she is free to make and no one has the right to judge her.

It will be tough. You'll have bad moments, maybe bad days. But take it all with a pinch of salt and make sure to get lots of pictures! These days will not come back. Appreciate what you have and be grateful for it. These things are possible only if you are surviving. If not, you'll be irritable, cranky and unhappy. You won't be a nice anybody, let alone a nice mom. So engage help. Take what breaks you can. Don't go on guilt trips. Start taking some time out for yourself and for each other. Hang in there. IT WILL GET BETTER. I promise.

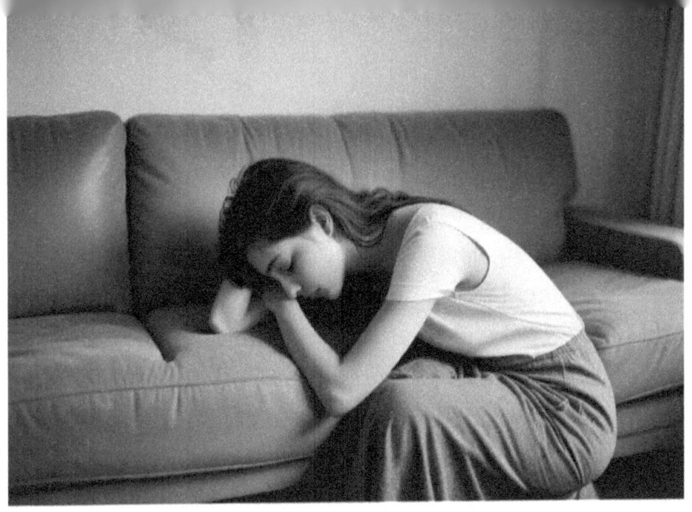

Chapter 22

POST-PARTUM BLUES

Kimaya has always been the poster girl for nature holding over nurture. She was born with genes that ensured she never put on weight and had that glass-like skin that we all think K-beauty rituals can give us. She didn't need to spend a rupee to get there and zilch effort to maintain her skinny yet wholesome figure while I was trying the GM diet and hitting a gym 6 days a week. She had Miraya 6 years after marriage, and her pregnancy was also a breeze. But, the same pregnancy left her with a really sagging tummy and horrible stretch marks. It also meant that she could no longer wear a lot of the kind of clothes that she had always preferred and had to buy a wardrobe that suited her new mommy bod. She spent a large part of the first days of her newborn staring at the mirror and secretly loathing the child she had once dreamt of holding because of what having Kimaya had done to her body.

While for ordinary mortals like me who have been dealing with things like this all life long, changes for the worse in my body after delivery were no big deal, for Kim, it was a life-altering experience. And one that she didn't handle well. It led her to spiral into post-partum depression, and she suddenly found herself obsessing over lotions and serums that promised to get rid of the loose skin and stretch marks. She started seeing flaws in her body where there were none. It was really terrible. It took almost 18 months of intense therapy to help her recover reasonably from the depression, and even then, it was a bit difficult for the acceptance to be complete. Fortunately, she stopped blaming the baby and realised that it was something most women go through. She also came to terms eventually with the fact that one can't maintain the same physical appearance through all phases of life. Although this kind of behaviour sounds ridiculous, it is something that women deal with in the aftermath of pregnancy whether they like it or not.

The first few weeks fly by in a blur. You may or may not remember many things barring a few rather significant incidents from that period. I certainly don't remember all the details. Eventually, you get so busy with the present of the child, even if it's not your first one, that your brain starts overwriting the space occupied by unimportant stuff with that which you really want to remember.

What you will, however, remember to some extent is your struggle. While it does get easier in a lot of ways, the battle is not necessarily easy. While not all of us go into what is categorically defined as 'post-partum depression,' most of us border on the verge and are usually kept on the border by some small saving grace or someone who helped us hang in there.

Throughout the book, I've stressed the value of relationships and making sure that the parents-to-be don't alienate themselves in the process of having a child. Believe me when I say it does take a village to raise a child. You cannot do it alone. If you've been trying it any other way, it's a mistake that's going to cost you in more ways than one.

Be careful through the process to put systems into place. Get people onboard who can be enlisted to help you, either because they care enough to help or just because they get paid for it. If you don't do this, it's going to be a tough battle. I've tried the hard way and I know.

When I conceived my eldest, we weren't living with the extended family. For a -4year period, we all lived in different apartment complexes in a -3kilometre radius and didn't necessarily help each other out. While I would meet the family occasionally, they weren't necessarily within reach when I needed help. Also, my husband and I had convinced ourselves that we were going to be the best parents possible only by being the most hands-on parents. While we had seen his sister relying significantly on paid help, we didn't feel that was how we wanted to be as parents. We were not the partying types or in a space in our careers where we needed to work long hours. We thought that between the 2 of us, and with the occasional help from his parents with whom we have always lived, we would be able to manage. It was a mistake.

When my baby was a little over 2 months old, I fell sick. I had a bout of flu, just a regular flu. Couldn't talk without sneezing and my body ached all over. Remember, I was also only just 2 months post-delivery. My husband had to stay home from work, and I hadn't started going to work yet. Four hours of coping with my feisty angel, and he'd had enough. I had already been dropping hints about wanting at least part-time help because once the baby starts turning, you can't leave her unattended. Unless she's one of those unusually quiet babies, if she senses she's alone, she's going to start bawling at the top of her lungs. So at least that was the case with mine. I couldn't go to the bathroom easily unless she was asleep, couldn't get extra baby-related chores done along with my regular workload, and definitely was in no position to resume working full-time. I'd been managing part-time work only just.

So yeah. This doesn't sound painful enough, but try it at your own risk. A cranky toddler who wants to be rocked to sleep in the parents' arms every single time. A sleep-deprived, cranky mother who's still recovering from baby birth and struggling to get all her work done. A father who's doing nighttime diaper and putting-the-baby-to-sleep duty to help his worn-out partner, barely hanging in there because he's got his plate full as well. Not good. Get help so that both of you don't wear yourselves out too fast and so that you can focus on the important thing rather than just go through the motions of raising your child. Do it before you've lost your senses in that quagmire of post-natal depression.

It's real. Just like any other ailment. Post-partum depression does exist, and it really takes its toll on someone who's learning how to be a new someone – a parent. It makes you feel inadequate and worthless and gives you such a tough time. You really don't know what hit you. This was supposed to all be magical and make your life so complete and full of joy. It does look complete on the outside and it's full, but full of stress and insecurities too. You can't do it alone, and if you don't have the help or the mental wherewithal required to really deal with the toughest of situations, don't even attempt it.

Avoid getting into the situation while you can. It is possible to plan better and build an organisation that is your set-up. Divide work, delegate responsibilities where you can, use gadgets and apps, keep the tempo going on things where you're replaceable. If you get your act together, you can have a better life post the arrival of your baby and you won't find yourself wanting. You can reduce the burden that you and your partner are going to deal with and make you save your energy for the things that matter the most to you. You don't have to prove a thing to ANYONE by doing it all yourself.

If you're living in the misbelief that you can prove a thing to anyone by being a lone warrior, firstly, let me tell you it's not worth it. People are going to point fingers and talk no matter what. If you get help, they'll call you lazy and irresponsible. If you don't get help, they'll call you stingy and stupid and still irresponsible. If your baby is fine and you're poorly turned out, they'll say you don't have to look like a rag to prove you're a good parent. If your baby is fine and you're well turned out, they'll say you probably leave the baby to the help all the time. They will talk either way.

God-forbid if your baby is on the skinny side, you're surely not breastfeeding her enough. If your baby is nice and chubby, you're probably ODing her on formula. If you've put on weight, surely you must not be feeding the baby or still eating for 2! If you're losing weight quickly, you must be starving yourself and imagine what kind of nutrition the baby must be getting. It's relentless, it's endless and you can never shut them up. So, just make sure you make the choices that put only one person at ease in their mind – yourself.

How your partner feels is definitely important but if he/she is not the primary caretaker of the child and is away for hours at a stretch, make sure to discuss what you want. If both of you are on the same page, great. If not, make sure to make your voice heard and put your interests on the same level as those of your child. An unhappy parent isn't going to make for a happy child. The child is supposed to be feeding off your body, not your soul.

I must point out here that there's no standard formula to parenting. No one size fits all. What works for me may or may not work for you. What works for you may not work for me. Every child is different and so is every parent and their circumstances. Therefore, you must figure out what it is that makes your family work and not get into a zone where you're only replicating the actions of others without gauging the impact on your life.

Oh, also, having a lot of everything without the time to manage anything isn't a good tactic. So try and practice caution when you shop for yourself and your baby during and after pregnancy. You don't want to bury yourself in a mountain of stuff that'll either never get used or get used only a couple of times and end up with fat credit card bills. The amount of noise by marketers on baby products is deafening and is very likely to drown your inner voice of wisdom while you buy. So be wise. Don't over-buy and overspend. It is also a common factor adding to post-partum stress and depression.

Your life is going to go through so much change. It's not necessary that you will adapt to those changes perfectly. It will take time for you to adjust and get yourself up to speed. So be kind to yourself and ask for help when you need it. Even a baby gets fed when it cries. No one is going to see through your charade of perfection and offer help unless you let them know what it is that you're really going through. It's possible you may not get the help you wanted, but then you can always try to find backups.

There are tons of online support groups that can give you quick answers to any tricky problems you face. At the same time, they may cause an information overload on your sensitive cranial hardware. Exercise caution and be careful in choosing what advice you follow and leave the rest out. Even after all this, if you do succumb to depression, seek professional help. There's no shame in it. As you would like to get help for a viral fever or a fracture or any other kind of problem, ask for help with managing your mind. It'll help you heal and be a better you.

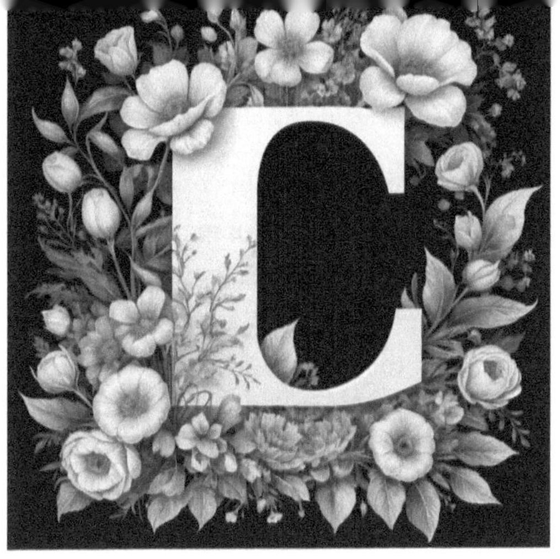

Chapter 23

PLAN C

We've spoken in depth about the options related to conception and assisted reproduction. It works out for most people. But there is an option for those for whom it didn't: adoption.

While there is an increasing number of people, singles and couples, who are opting to adopt a child, there is a lot of stigma around it as well. There are those who will say that nurture can never win over nature and that one's own blood will always be one's own blood and whatnot. Please understand that adoption is a choice not of having a child alone, but it's a beautiful act where everyone wins. A child without a home gets a family to call his own and at the same time, a family that had been wanting a child, gets to have one to bring up as their own.

Let me also clarify that I have not adopted a child. I have 3 biological ones. I admire those who have done it and at some point in time, dreamt of doing it myself one day. But after having 3 kids, I'm not sure I'm ready for the responsibility of another. I don't think I got the opportunity to even seriously plan for it or to consider it because my kids were conceived in such quick succession, and I didn't have the desire to go in for an abortion at any point because there was no real reason to not have the baby I was carrying. That's my life. Your life may be significantly different from mine and your choices would depend on how your life is panning out.

At the same time, I know enough families that have adopted a child after having had one biologically or even 2. I really, really do admire them and wish them the best in the world. It's a choice that you should also consider yourself fortunate enough to have. To be able to choose to become a parent in such a way and to bring a child in need of a home into yours and give them everything you can, is not just a really noble act, it's also the purest form of love possible. Simply because you chose to do it. I'm not saying having an adopted child is better or anything than having a biological one, but that you choose to do it is a fabulous thing.

If all else fails, or if you succeeded and want a bigger family, by all means go out there and let a child into your home. You will both be blessed and your life will be wonderful for it. It's not a choice for those without one. It's a choice that only those who truly want to love can make. Because it doesn't matter to them where the object of their affection came from and how he/she came to be where they were. All that matters is that someone who deserves to be loved gets the love that they deserve.

This book has been full of all kinds of stories. I wish I could've shared so many more with you. Because each person who has had a baby or who's trying to have one has such a different one to tell. Everyone goes through different things because each one's life is different. Which story may have struck a chord with you, I can't tell, but I hope something would've found a mark.

In the process of this book, I've tried to help you not only prepare yourself for the process of becoming a parent, but also your partner and those around you so that you can all welcome the child with open arms. To have a baby is a beautiful thing. It cannot be described adequately in words. But it comes with such a mountain of responsibility and with so many complications that cannot be wished away.

So if you've read this book with an open mind, you'll find that you can learn a lot from my experiences and those of my friends and family, and make your life easier. I'm not saying it will be perfect if you do. Not at all. But at least you've had some amount of forewarning and can plan for the things that many other people before you never had the opportunity to know about beforehand.

Plans don't always work out. We plan because we're optimistic. But we must be realistic and learn to adapt to the situation if our original plans don't work out. That's why we have a plan B and a plan C. You don't know what life has in store for you, so try one thing at a time. If you're fortunate, you'll get what you want the way you want it. If not, you must only reset your thinking to acknowledge that you didn't know what you needed and be grateful to have gotten what you needed instead of what you wanted. After all, what we want is not always what we need.

Your relationship with your child, like any other relationship in life, will also go through its share of ups and downs. While you may have prepared yourself for what it will take for you to have the baby itself, how you're going to eventually deal with the baby herself is a different question altogether.

Perhaps someday, you and I can have a conversation about that too. Till then, all the best with your quest for a child. May you have a wonderful pregnancy and a healthy, happy child!